by Dr. N. W. Walker

The Natural Way To Vibrant Health

Norwalk PRESS

Printed in Canada

Published by Norwalk Press
An imprint of Book Publishing Company
PO Box 99
Summertown, TN 38483
(888) 260-8458
www.bookpubco.com

ISBN 10: 0-89019-035-6
ISBN 13: 978-0-89019-035-7

In publishing this book, it is not Dr. Walker's or the Publisher's intent to diagnose or prescribe, but only to inform the reader. Dr. Walker recommends the reader contact a professional doctor specializing in the appropriate subject.

Book Publishing Co. is a member of Green Press Initiative. We chose to print this title on paper with postconsumer recycled content, processed without chlorine, which saved the following natural resources:

252 pounds of solid waste   9 trees
861 pounds of greenhouse gases
4,147 gallons of water   3 million BTU of energy

For more information, visit <www.greenpressinitiative.org>. Savings calculations from the Environmental Defense Paper Calculator, <www.edf.org/papercalculator>.

You don't need to relate your health to your age! For more than 100 years, Norman W. Walker, Ph.D., proved through research that well-being and long life can go hand-in-hand. Modern day nutritionists and medical researchers are just now discovering the truths which Dr. Walker has known and, expounded throughout the twentieth century. Dr. Walker himself was living proof that a longer, healthier life may be achieved through proper diet, mental soundness, and intelligent body care. Every year we read about a new fad diet, a "cure-all" drug, a food supplement, or a revolutionary exercise program that will save our lives. The Dr. Walker program is unique in that it doesn't use the promotional words, "miracle, fad, or revolutionary" . . . it doesn't need them!

Dr. Walker's contributions to our living longer, healthier lives began before the turn of the century in London, where as a young man he became seriously ill from over-work. Unable to accept the idea of ill health or a sick body, Dr. Walker cured himself. Since that time, he spent the balance of his life searching man's ability to extend life and achieve freedom from disease.

In 1910, Dr. Walker established the Norwalk Laboratory of Nutritional Chemistry and Scientific Research in New York, and thus began his important contributions to a longer, more active form of living. Among his great contributions, was the discovery of the therapeutic, value of fresh vegetable juices, and in 1930 the development of the Triturator Juicer.

We believe Dr. Walker was one of the world's leading nutritionist; his unique contributions are all available to you through his books.

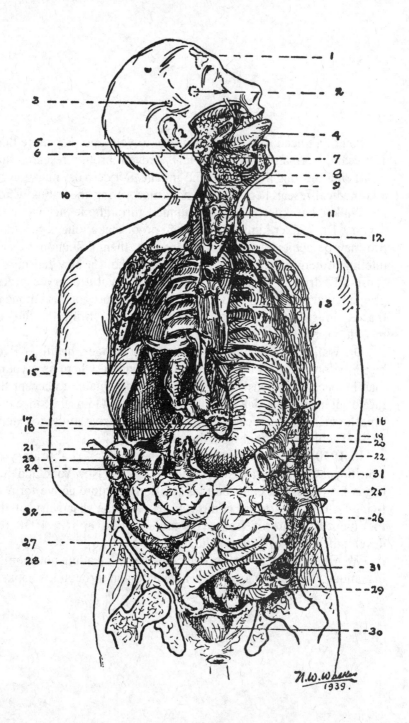

It is my opinion that the most important subject missing in elementary schools, is ANATOMY.

This sketch is included here to serve as a guide and handy reference.

The numbers indicate the location of the various parts.

1. The Frontal Sinus, in the forehead, above the eye where mucus accumulates eventually when we eat excessive amounts of concentrated starches, and drink too much milk.

2. The Pituitary Gland (or Body) is located directly behind and just a little below the level of the bridge of the nose.

3. The Pineal Gland, located in the mid-brain, back, and slightly higher than the Pituitary.

4. The Tongue, one of the most mischievous organs of the human body.

5. The Medulla Oblongata, the central Nerve-telephone-exchange, is situated in the lower middle part of the head, between the upper lip and the base of the skull, just above the Atlas or first cervical vertebra.

6. The Parotid Gland, which becomes swollen and causes Mumps, especially when children and adolescents indulge in excesses of starches and candies.

7. The Sub-Lingual Gland.

8. Sub-Maxillary Gland.

9. The Epiglottis.

10. The Pharynx

11. The Thyroid Gland, one of the most vital and important glands of the body. It requires Iodine-foods for proper functioning. When improperly nourished causes Goiter.

12. The Larynx.

13. The Spleen is located towards the back of number 19. Back of the Ribs at this point are the Lungs; back of the Lungs, the Stomach the Splenic Flexure of the Colon, the Spleen, the tip of the Pancreas and the left Kidney.

14. The Gall Bladder - That most essential, though greatly abused gland. The Liver (No. 15) has been raised in this picture, with a hook, to show its location. Its duct leads into the Duodenum (No. 24) to lubricate the intestines with the bile. To remove a Gall Bladder (instead of cleansing the system naturally) deprives the unlucky individual of Nature's means for lubricating the intestines sufficiently.

15. The Liver - The most marvelous laboratory in Creation. Created by Nature to withstand on an average about 40 to 50 years of abuse after birth before perceptible and usually uncomfortable disintegration begins.

16. The Stomach - That organ which controls the Individual, unless the Individual learns to control it.

17. The Pyloric Valve, between the Stomach and Duodenum.
18. The Pancreas , the gland which enables the body to utilize natural sugars (such as are found in raw fruits and vegetables) and which breaks down when refined sugars and starches are used to excess causing diabetes.
19. The Splenic Flexure of the Colon, or the bend in the Colon leading from the Transverse Colon (No. 22 and No. 23) to the Descending Colon (No. 31).
20. The general location (further back) of the Kidneys.
21. The Hepatic Flexure of the Colon, leading from the Ascending Colon (No. 32) to the Transverse Colon (Nos. 23-22).
22. The Transverse Colon, frequently becomes a gas storage balloon when
23. tense nerves or impactions of waste matter in the Flexures (Nos. 21-29) prevent the gas from expanding and being expelled. As a result of improper nourishment this section of the Colon easily loses its tone and then sags, causing what is more picturesquely described as a prolapsus.
24. The Duodenum, or Second Stomach, where the alkaline digestive processes we so frequently interfered with by the presence of acid or acid-forming foods with concentrated starches and sugars, often resulting in ulcerous conditions which individuals enjoy calling their Duodenal Ulcers.
25. The area of the Solar Plexus.
26. The Small Intestines, about 25 feet of perpetual trouble, sooner or later, for those who insist on eating what they want when they want it.
27. The Appendix, that marvelous safety gland whose secretion prevents gas-forming bacteria and other noxious germs from passing into the Small Intestines from the Colon. It has of late been allowed to function more normally since the education of the laity in the use of frequent enemas and skillful colonic irrigations.
28. The Bladder is in this region.
29. The Sigmoid Flexure of the Colon leading from the Descending Colon (No. 31) to the Rectum (No. 30).
30. The Rectum, the cesspool of the body, which should be washed out with enemas or colonic irrigations quite often.
31. The Descending Colon.
32. The Ascending Colon.

CONTENTS.

CONTENTS.
(Continued)

Chapter 1
START HERE:

This is strictly personal - for YOU!

The quick, rapid change of a life habit or pattern may be disastrous. To attain **VIBRANT HEALTH** is not an over-night process.

I truly believe you will find this the most up-to-date yet timeless volume in your collection of books.

Here you will discover that mysterious power that changes lives, that ennobles the spirit, that broadens the vision, that enriches the mind and stimulates your aspirations.

This book is not for the general public. It is written intentionally as a very personal volume for YOU. My objective is to help you to attain **VIBRANT HEALTH** by perceiving your goals in life, by comprehending your problems and your future in relation to your health and environment.

This book is not intended to be a scholastic treatise expounding scientific technical theories propounded with profuse quotations from the writings of other authors. On the contrary, it is imbued with the basic principles which I have proven from my own practice and experience, which have led me to attain and to maintain **VIBRANT HEALTH.**

If this publication succeeds in guiding you to explore more deeply this fabulous mine of spiritual, mental and health treasures and values, I will have accomplished my aim.

I am placing the whole subject before you, shall I say, as my secret, divulged to you as one seeker after THE TRUTH, to another, without condemnation or criticism of anybody or anything. It is by no means intended as an argumentative dissertation for discussion. I have endeavored, rather, to demonstrate and to prove to you that, having found THE POSSIBLE DREAM to become a reality as have thousands of others, you, too, can achieve **VIBRANT HEALTH!**

Chapter 2
WHY SHOULD YOU WANT
VIBRANT HEALTH?

VIBRANT HEALTH is the indisputable foundation for the satisfaction of a life more abundant.

The present tempo of living, the rate of pressure and speed which regulates the present daily span of our life, would be incomprehensible to any who lived back in the 1900's, and if suddenly brought into present day living, they would be unable to cope with it.

The problem which faces us today is to find a way to try to live to be healthy in order to keep up a speed of existence unheard of a century ago.

Today, in spite of everything "modernized" and more or less streamlined, most people just THINK they are healthy because they can say: "Oh, I'm O.K., I'm fine, I have no specific complaints".

As a matter of fact there is a vast gulf between just feeling O.K. with no specific ailments, and experiencing **VIBRANT HEALTH**. If all false stimulants such as tobacco, alcohol beverages, soft drinks, coffee, drugs, etc., were suddenly unavailable, I have often wondered how many people would collapse!

These people have no concept of what **VIBRANT HEALTH** is, that kind of health that makes one feel literally intoxicated with LIFE, with the urge to do and to be beyond the capacity and limitations of any day's efforts, with untiring energy, clarity of mind, unquenchable enthusiasm. One cannot possibly realize how WONDERFUL it is to have **VIBRANT HEALTH**, without actually experiencing it.

Rarely do we find an individual so VIBRANTLY HEALTHY that he bubbles over, who is fairly bursting with ambition and enthusiasm, pulsating with energy, effervescing with vitality.

Are YOU one of these individuals?

If you do not happen to be such a remarkable person, DO you want to be one? You CAN! All it takes is "know-how", perseverance and stick-to-itivness. This should be your goal in life, to be VIBRANTLY HEALTHY, full of vim, vigor and vitality of the supreme soul-satisfying kind.

YOU CAN DO IT!

Chapter 3
DO YOU KNOW HOW OLD I AM?

By and large, the present younger generation already seems to be beginning to look and act prematurely old, judging by their dress and appearance.

As I pass school buildings, when classes are over and the children are leaving for home, I observe young girls, even under 10 years of age, going home from school dressed in long old fashioned dresses which were the vogue a hundred years ago, dresses so long that sometimes they have to hold them up to keep from tripping over their skirts.

What a strange mixed up age we are living in! One cannot tell the boys from the girls by their appearance, nor can one discern their age. Some of these youngsters already look like old men and women.

Obviously this young generation is not at all age-conscious. Regardless how they appear, however, they all seem to be seeking a better way of life. To me they seem to be a very intelligent generation of young people seeking TRUTH wherever they can find it. They really want answers to their multitude of questions.

This is very gratifying to me, because since my first book was published back in the 1930's it has been mostly older people who purchased my books and were interested in better health. Now the trend seems to be completely reversed.

Imagine a 17 year old girl writing to me recently that she was so happy to discover my book **BECOME YOUNGER** because she was very much interested in BECOMING YOUNGER! Every mail brings me letters from these young people, intelligent, happy, enthusiastic letters telling me how much they have enjoyed my books, which they say have opened up a whole new way of life for them.

I can truly say that these letters have given me a completely new lease on life and I have begun writing again! It is my deepest desire to give any guidance and help I can to these bright, inquiring young people. Since it is impossible for me to answer even a fraction of the letters I receive, I hope this book and my other publications will help to guide them, if they will take the time to study them.

Do not EVER tell anybody how old you are! Once people know how many years have slipped under the bridge of your life since you first set foot on it, your name will go into a pigeon-hole and that-will-be-that! The number of years you have spent or misspent in this physical body do not indicate your stature. It is how you live and what you accomplish, without ever thinking how old you are, that will enable you to be AGELESS after four or five score years or more.

I can truthfully say that I am never conscious of my age. Since I reached maturity I have never been aware of being any older, and I can say, without equivocation or mental reservation, that I feel more alive, awake, alert and full of enthusiasm today than I did when I was 30 years old. I still feel that my best years are ahead of me.

I never think of birthdays, nor do I celebrate them. Today I can truthfully say that I am enjoying **VIBRANT HEALTH,** I don't mind telling people how old I am: I AM AGELESS!

A classic example of the reason for not acknowledging your chronological age struck me very forcefully while I was listening to the tape recording of a talk by a friend who recently was fitted with glasses. In the middle of his talk he said: "I just can't get accustomed to these bifocals. I had a new pair of glasses fitted and the optometrist told me that, because I was 40 years old, I SHOULD have bifocals. I didn't think I needed them, but he said I did, because I was 40 years old".

How ridiculous! This is one reason why I am opposed to telling my chronological age. Everywhere one goes today, whether seeking employment, to the dentist, optometrist or doctor, it is the same thing — they ask you how old you are and then immediately they put you in a pigeon-hole and there you remain for the rest of your days. They have a special classification grouping for every age bracket.

Physical, mental and spiritual qualities should be considered first. I definitely object to this mass-type analysis.

I am in complete possession of my faculties and I am alive, alert, energetic and full of enthusiasm. How old am I?? I AM AGELESS!

Chapter 4
THINK VIBRANT HEALTH

"As a man thinketh in his heart, so is he." (Proverbs 23-7)

Dr. Norman Vincent Peale (In volume 23, No. I part III of his "Creative Help for Daily Living" pamphlet) records his conversation with the young driver of the Motel's courtesy car, when leaving Chicago to return to New York.

"How are you feeling this morning?" The young driver asked Dr. Peale, who answered: I'm pretty good".

"Pretty good! The driver exclaimed, Pretty good isn't enough".

"Well, said Dr. Peale, how are you?"

"I am just great (answered the young man) I'm terrific! I haven't got an unhealthy thought in my head. I think well and I am well".

The chauffeur is quoted as telling Dr. Peale:

"You often tell people that the way to feel healthy is to think healthy. You're right! A long time ago I made up my mind to practice being vital and alive".

Dr. Peale continues in his article: "Now there is always somebody ready to argue about the idea that thinking and practicing healthy thoughts can make you well. They will say: 'But I've got something really wrong with me'. We do not minimize organic disease at all, but even if there is something wrong, the forces of vitality and health can still be stimulated by how you think".

I agree perfectly with Dr. Peale, and I am one hundred percent in accord with the fact that, as you express the state of your condition, so it reacts both on you and on your listeners. I never fail to get an uplift and much satisfaction from the reaction of people who ask me "How are you?" My answer is invariably: "I'm right on top of the world!" Even the gloomiest individual who is exposed to my answer, whether he is my questioner or a bystander, will crack his face into a smile which continues to remain after I have left. If you want to feel that uplift, try telling people: "Oh, I am right on top of the world!", and FEEL it while you are saying it. Your gloomiest thoughts will instantly vanish!

The clarity with which young people are summing up our present day problems was brought out clearly to my mind when I received a long letter from a young married man from whom I have received no word for a long time. He writes, and I quote:

"In the past couple of years, conditions in the world have caused me to rethink many things. We have done a good bit of traveling over the world the past few years, having lived in various urban areas, and have seen much of the moral decay of our societies. It would seem to me that man is very much headed down a dead-end road. The century-old 'man-is-god' theory (that if we put enough man, money, energy and priorities to any problem, man can solve it and at the same time create a utopia), is certainly disproving itself.

"Our problems seem to be doubling the rate that solutions are coming; and people everywhere are searching for meaning and purpose in life. It is from these feelings that we decided to make the move to ... and give up our "great dreams". If things are going to change, we thought maybe we should start with ourselves".

What perspicacity and intelligence comes from this young man!

This is still another confirmation that young people are searching, and searching, and searching for the secret of an abundant life, health, and a purpose to exist more completely. In other words: in **VIBRANT HEALTH.**

Chapter 5
SEEK!
AND YOU SHALL FIND

Some months ago I was introduced to a successful Engineer and I mean successful. He looked me over, as I thought, to appraise me, then made this remarkable statement:

"Dr. Walker, I am glad to meet you, but you are not at all what I expected to see!"

"Oh," I said, "what could you possibly expect to see in me"

"Well, I expected to see a more portly and imposing man. You are much too thin to be a good example for your teachings. Now, I weigh just about 325 pounds and I am healthy and strong, with never a sick day. Judging by your frame, you should be much heavier !"

"Oh?," I replied, "you never have a headache, heartburn, indigestion, liver trouble? Did you ever see a fat race horse? I am of the race horse type and am never troubled with any of these disturbances."

"Ah," he countered, "but these are natural conditions which everybody is subject to!"

"Oh no, indeed," I exclaimed, "if you were to lose 100 or 125 pounds it would not take you long to realize that these "natural" conditions are, literally, indications of a sick body. Just give this angle a thought."

I met this same gentleman a week or two ago and I hardly recognized him. He told me that as soon as we parted the last time we met, he went to a Health Food Store and bought all my books and read them through.

"They made sense," he said, and he started immediately first with a series of colon irrigations, then eliminating from his meals, gradually, what was indicated as not constructive. His weight was down to 210 pounds, with no more of these "conditions which are natural and to which everybody is subject"

And just at this point I was interrupted by a long distance telephone call from a young woman with a sweet voice, who was perplexed because her friends just did not understand how she could follow our Program, and be healthy.

She asked me: What do you do for a headache? I said: I don't have any. She replied that she rarely did, but some of her friends have them and wanted her to ask me what to do. I told her that if I ever

7

should have one, the very first thing I would do would be to clean out the system and the headaches would follow suit.

I want to tell you that, in spite of their long hair and appearance, these young people are just too precious for words. They are all seeking the TRUTH, so anxious to know what is right for them to do, and they are keenly interested in following only what will give them a better and healthier life. They come from all walks of life. They ask such intelligent questions and - they follow through.

Chapter 6
IMPROVING MIND AND POWER.

Did you ever notice a sick dog, or a sick cat, or a sick calf? They are such pitiful things!

Did you ever give some thought to how frustrated YOU can be, when you yourself are sick?

When you are sick you can't even think straight!

Do you realize what that means, that you can't even THINK STRAIGHT?

Thinking and Health go hand in hand, and I can vouch for that from my personal experience. So, when I am writing about **VIBRANT HEALTH** I am covering a subject regarding which I am well qualified to write.

There are many degrees of Health. There is that sense of being well enough to say: "Oh, I'm pretty well".

Or there may be that sense of health that leads one to say: "I'd feel fine if it were not for that confounded pain in my joints!"

Another one may say: "I've just come from my doctor's and he tells me there is nothing wrong with me. I just wish he could feel the way I do right now, then his story would be quite different!"

These people are sick, but they don't know it. They lack what it takes to experience VIBRANT HEALTH!

Do you, for one moment, think that any of these people, when asked: "How are you today?" can honestly answer: "I am right on top of the world?"

No, they cannot, because in the present state of their consciousness their mind is warped by concentration on ill-health.

Do you think that any of these people can have their mind and their spirit so well attuned to their highest potential that they can sail through their days filled with peace of mind, happiness and the general state that can only be experienced when we have **VIBRANT HEALTH?**

No, they cannot do so for the very same reason. They cannot concentrate on a positive plane of thought while the mind is immovably centered on negative and disruptive concepts.

There are many cliches which contain more truth than fiction, such as:

You are what you eat.

You are what you think.

You are as old - or as young - as you think you are, etc.

The root of all these epigrammatic maxims lies in every phase of your existence, in your emotional state, in the food you eat, and in the extent that waste matter is eliminated from your body.

When I expound on clarity of intellect, on the power of the mind, on the state of consciousness that places one on that higher plane of understanding that broadens one's perspective, that expands one's perceptions, and that sharpens one's intelligence, I expound on these because experience and observation have proven to me that through **VIBRANT HEALTH** all these are possible.

Food and the state of mind work hand in hand. The very best food becomes a poison in the system when negative emotions are present during eating. When one is tired, angry, worried, fearful, jealous, or in any other such state of consciousness, one should refrain from eating or drinking anything, until one can become rested and calm. To put food in the system at such negative times causes unpredictable reactions, the food does not digest properly and the result is toxemia.

On the other hand, when a happy, gay, cheerful, joyful, sunny atmosphere prevails during a meal, even little things that might otherwise annoy one, are readily overlooked and discounted, so that the meal is a pleasant affair and the digestion responds in kind and quality. The entire alimentary tract becomes buoyant and responsive, while at the same time the eliminative organs are ready to take care of the waste material that needs to be eliminated and removed from the body. The result is the assimilation of food in the best accepted manner.

By enjoying one's meal the entire emotional reactions are constructive and conducive to the improvement of the mind, with energy and power for the body.

At every meal, hold this thought in your mind: I WANT **VIBRANT HEALTH,** AND I'M GOING TO GET IT! then smile or laugh, because the most powerful digestive agent in the world is YOUR OWN SMILE OF CONTENTMENT AND ENJOYMENT when you are eating your dinner or any other meal!

Chapter 7
THE ATTENTION
YOUR BODY NEEDS.

When you seriously undertake the steps necessary to regenerate your physical body, you become aware of the ease with which one slips into the negative line of least resistance in the matter of nutrition, with no concern as to the kind and quality of the food one eats. You look around, and you wonder how people have managed to live as long as they do on the destructive diets and other undeniably noxious foods and beverages used to appease the appetite. You wonder how people can exist with so little attention given to bodily needs.

The reason for such survival lies in the foresight of our Creator in supplying the human body with such a miraculous surplus of expendable material (material that is constantly used up and replenished) which is necessary for the regeneration of the cells and tissues of the body. The material which I have called expendable consists of the atoms which compose the cells with which the human body is built.

The number of atoms in your body is beyond your ability to calculate them, yet each atom is virtually a self contained universe enclosing a terrific amount of energy and power. It is the life-principle in these infinitely microscopic atoms that makes it possible for you to be what you are.

Your body is the house in which you live. By analogy it is just like the building in which you make your home. Your home needs, at the very least, periodical attention, otherwise the roof may leak, the plumbing will get out of order and get clogged up, termites will drill through the floors and the walls, and other innumerable cases of deterioration will make their appearance.

Such is the case with your physical body. Every function and activity of your system, day and night, physical, mental and spiritual, is dependent on the attention you give to your body.

Consider, for example, the operation of your Endocrine Glands. These Endocrine Glands must have compatible conditions of nutrition, of intercommunication one with another, and of cleanliness, otherwise their efficiency is impaired. The energy which enables these Endocrine Glands to operate comes from the atoms composing them, together with the atoms composing the nutrition upon which they are fed. Namely, the food you eat. The importance of these Endocrine Glands is appreciated when you realize that they are involved in every function and activity of your body.

The kind and the quality of the food is of vital importance to every phase of your existence. Nutrition not only regenerates and rebuilds the cells and tissues which constitute your physical body, but also is involved in the processes by which the waste matter, the undigested food, is eliminated from your body to prevent corruption in the form of fermentation and putrefaction in the body. This corruption and putrefaction, if retained and allowed to accumulate in the body prevents any possibility of attaining any degree of **VIBRANT HEALTH.**

It is both important and vital for you to beware of the type of food which your body needs to nourish it. If the type of food is correct and constructive, your body will respond by supplying you with an abundant amount of energy, vigor and vitality, physically; and will enable your mind and emotions to help you to be in control of life instead of letting life control you, as would otherwise be the case with improper and incompatible foods.

Bear in mind that a home or residence built of brick, stone or wood, or other material, when neglected beyond the advisability to repair it, can be torn down and replaced by another one. Not so with your body. If you neglect your body to the point of no return, you cannot discard it and buy a new one to replace it.

A body may appear to be in perfect health, from outward appearances, but remember—the body starts falling apart from the inside. By the time there is an outward manifestation that all is not well, it may even then be too late to repair or rebuild it. Like a house which, to all appearances, is solid, firm and in perfect condition; actually it may really be eaten up by termites inside the floors and walls to the point of collapsing at any point under stress. A friend of ours one morning walked into her kitchen when, suddenly, the termite-eaten floor gave way beneath her. What a shock!!!! She was not overweight, either, and she had no idea, prior to this, that there were any termites in the house!

Do not be misled by outward appearances. The finest looking watch in the world is of no value if the main spring is defective. The most gorgeous luscious appearing apple will shock you if you cut it in half and find worms and rot in the core. The human body is no exception. Appearance alone is not an indication of health and certainly not of **VIBRANT HEALTH. VIBRANT HEALTH** is the reflection of perfect harmony within the entire system, of every gland and every organ in the body properly nourished and kept consistently cleansed. My purpose in writing this book is to alert you on these facts and to inspire you to do something about your own condition.

Chapter 8
HOW I DISCOVERED
VIBRANT HEALTH
THROUGH FRESH RAW JUICES.

Today, as I am typing this manuscript, I am blessed with **VIBRANT HEALTH** - but it was not always so! As a matter of fact, the doctor told my parents, when I was about five years old, that he had done everything possible and that there was not a ghost of a chance that I would live out the night.

Let me digress, at this point, and relate three particular pertinent episodes in my life which have a definite and distinct bearing on the subject matter of this book, namely: **VIBRANT HEALTH.**

The Doctor Said I Was As Good As DEAD!

When I was about five years old I became afflicted with a fatal sickness, and I never did learn what it was. I became unconscious and fell into a coma. When I opened my eyes I saw my father and my mother kneeling at my bedside talking to God. I had the impression that my father was thanking God that they had been privileged to have me in the family for the past few years, and he beseeched God to recover my life and to restore my health.

I remember my father adding: "Heavenly Father, if it is Thy Will. . . ." Of course I did not know then what it was all about, nor what that meant, but that sentence so impressed itself on my consciousness that I have never forgotten it.

I said: "Mother, I'm thirsty". Eventually my mother told me that they both looked at me in surprise and astonishment. Sobbing, she brought me a warm drink. I later wondered why my Mother had cried when I had recovered, and that was my first introduction to the realization that no male can understand what a female does, and why!

Anyway, I recovered quickly, and when the doctor came the next day to see what he expected to be my corpse, he was utterly astounded to see me in my nightgown standing in front of the window, looking out, totally unconcerned about anything else. This I have remembered ever since. Now you know why I believe in miracles!

My childhood and youthful adolescence were those of a boy who must be watched that he does not overdo. You know how that is.

That was my first bout with Health.

In later years, after leaving home, I took a vacation and went to Belgium. One morning, while strolling through the Municipal Park in the City of Brussels, I came upon a scene of unforgettable beauty. The sun was streaming through a grove of pine trees, over magnificent huge ferns. I took a snapshot of the scene with my 35mm pocket Kodak and when I returned to England I had the film developed. I stared in joy and amazement at the beautiful 35mm photograph.

A Budding Artist - and I lost sleep.

The vivid recollection of the actual scene inspired me to buy a sheet of Watman's drawing paper big enough to enable me to draw an enlargement of the 35 mm snapshot to about 11½ by 17 ½ inches. I also bought a bottle of India drawing ink, a very fine lithographic pen and a magnifying glass.

That night, after dinner, I set to work in my bedroom and began to draw the picture, working from about 7 until 2 or 3 o'clock in the morning. This continued night after night for a WHOLE NINE MONTHS, notwithstanding the fact that I had to go to the office from 9 a.m. till. 5 p.m. at least five days a week.

This loss of rest and sleep did me no harm—so I thought, in my young smug conceit. However, I had the satisfaction of sending the finished picture to my mother for her birthday. Upon her demise I confiscated the picture and presented it to my precious wife. Now it hangs on the wall in our living room, over our Hammond Organ.

But that is only the beginning of the story.

I Was A Nervous Wreck

About three years later I was actively engaged in a business of my own when, out of the blue (as the saying is) I was stricken with a serious nervous breakdown. My doctor told me that my liver was grievously involved. He advised me to forget all my affairs in England, if I wanted to try to get better, and to go to the North of France, where he was sure I would find some farmers who would feed me solely from the products of their garden.

I promptly packed my things and went into Brittany, on the Northwest coast of France. After a couple of days or so, thanks to my ability to speak French fluently, I did find an elderly French couple on their farm some distance from the village, not very far from the town of Pontivy on the Aulne River in the hills of Brittany. They were agreeable to have me as their paying guest - at the equivalent of about $2.00 a week for room and board! They ate only vegetables, mostly raw, and fruits from their garden, during the week. On Sundays they killed one of their roosters or a duck.

One morning I happened to go into the kitchen while the old lady was peeling carrots for lunch. Watching her, I noticed how moist these carrots were when peeled, although they had not yet been in water. That set my brain into high gear and I did some thinking. That afternoon I asked her permission to pick a few carrots and to peel them. And could I use her feed grinder? I set to work grinding about half a dozen good sized carrots, and by straining the pulp through one of her nice clean dish towels I obtained my first introduction to a cupful of beautiful carrot juice!

I made as much carrot juice each day as I could drink. The old folks also took to it.

My English Doctor had told me that it would take a long time, probably nine months or a year for me to get well. However, in about eight weeks I was back in England being examined by my very much amazed and astounded Doctor.

What is the corollary of the foregoing narrations?

In the first place, I started with a weak, unhealthy body, a veritable handicap. Howbeit, by the acquisition and application of knowledge I have been able to build my body into a VIBRANT HEALTHY condition.

In the second place, by my lack of rest and insufficient sleep I had succeeded in devitalizing my body to the point of being the easy victim of a very serious nervous breakdown.

Sleep And Rest-

Over the years I have been deeply impressed by the vast number of ailments which failed to come under the stereotyped classification of diagnoses.

Upon investigation I found that the contributing factor of perhaps ninety per cent of these ailments was the result of these patients having been so preoccupied with the vicissitudes of daily pressures at home and in business that they failed to take the time necessary to get the sleep that the human body MUST HAVE, and the essential amount of rest without which the human system slowly but surely begins to degenerate.

The basic principles of acquiring **VIBRANT HEALTH** consist of sufficient sleep and rest, conquering worry, anxiety, and all such negative states, and taking the proper care of nourishing the body and keeping it regularly cleansed inside as well as on the outside.

16

Juices For Health-

In the third place, my affliction and the consequent circumstances opened up the way for me to discover fresh raw vegetable and fruit juices and the means by which I have been able to build up and to maintain, for years on end, the degree of **VIBRANT HEALTH** that has brought me almost unbounded energy, vigor and vitality.

Chapter 9
THE WHY
OF FRESH RAW JUICES

My extensive studies in the Healing Arts gave me the clue to the successful steps necessary to develop and to maintain **VIBRANT HEALTH** by means of the various fresh raw vegetable juices.

That clue indicated to me that when we eat solid food it MUST be broken down by the digestive processes into liquids. This is necessary in order that these digestive processes may separate the atoms and molecules from the fibers to enable the atoms and molecules to pass, by osmosis, through the walls of the intestines. They can then be transported by the blood to the liver for reconversion into the type and kind of nutrients that the cells and tissues of the body need.

Fresh raw juices relieve the digestive system of much of the energy required to liquefy solid food. Solid food requires, on an average, from three to five hours to digest, whereas the juices are digested in a matter of minutes and they are assimilated into the system in a very few minutes more.

Osmosis is the chemical and physiological diffusion through the walls of the intestines of substances broken down and liquefied from a solid or semi-solid state into their atomic components. It is only in this "liberated" liquid state that the food components are able to enter the body through the walls of the intestines. They are then transported by the blood to the liver for reconstruction into the kind and type of nutrients that the cells and tissues of the body require.

What cannot be so liquefied in the digestive processes is eliminated as waste through the colon.

Now, do not jump to the conclusion that we should live solely on juices, eating no solid food. That would be neither logical nor sensible.

We DO need to eat plenty of fresh raw solid food, particularly in the form of vegetables, fruits, nuts and seeds and their sprouts, because their fibers are needed as roughage to act as an intestinal broom, figuratively speaking, so that the colon can have fibrous material to assist its movement to expel the waste products from the body. This is covered in my book **DIET & SALAD SUGGESTIONS.**

I consider fresh raw vegetable and fruit juices essential supplements to every meal — and an important part in the foundation for **VIBRANT HEALTH.**

Chapter 10
DIGESTION OF FOOD, AND
ELIMINATION OF WASTE.

Digestion presupposes the result of eating, and everybody knows that if we do not eat, we die.

Not everybody realizes, however, that failure to eliminate waste products from the body causes so much fermentation and putrefaction in the large intestine, or colon, that the neglected accumulation of such waste can, and frequently does, result in a lingering demise!

So, if we do not eat, we die, and if we do not cleanse our body, we may die prematurely, therefore both these conditions and their importance must be considered in the program to attain VIBRANT HEALTH - and to LIVE.

The elimination from the body of undigested food and of other waste products is equally as important as is the proper digestion and assimilation of food. In fact I can think of nothing more significant and vital, because of the danger of the inevitable effects of toxemia, of toxic poisons, as the outcome of the neglected accumulation and failure to expel feces, debris and other waste matter from the body.

Digestion is the essential process by means of which nutrients in the food you eat are assimilated by your body. Naturally, if food is not properly digested it cannot be completely assimilated and the body is deprived of needed nourishment; at least part of its nutrition is wasted.

Such waste must necessarily be expelled from the body, and for this purpose you are equipped with a very efficient eliminative sewage system, your colon. That is to say, "efficient" IF it is in good and proper working order functioning on the schedule suited to your physical condition.

Time It Takes For Food To Travel Through The Body-

Once food is taken into the mouth to be eaten, it must travel very slowly through some 25 feet of the alimentary canal. It takes an average from three to five hours before this passage is completed from the mouth to the end of the small intestine. Try walking a distance of 25 feet consuming 3 to 5 hours doing so and you will get the picture very clearly.

The small intestine ends at the Ileo-cecal valve, where the large intestine, or colon, begins. The residue which leaves the small intestine at this juncture passes on into the colon, which should normally measure about five feet in length. If the colon is clean and is functioning naturally and normally, it will take another hour or two for the feces to pass through to the rectum for its expulsion through the anus.

Safety Valve —
The Ileo-cecal valve is the safety valve where the small intestine joins the colon. It is located in the region of the right groin. Its purpose is to control the speed of the passage of residue through it, while at one and the same time to prevent any matter or substance from returning back into the small intestine from the colon.

While it functions normally the chances are that the digestive system is either in good condition or that there may not be too much wrong with it. If the colon clogs up it means TROUBLE!

Study sketch.

The ileo-cecal valve is equipped with a safety mechanism which opens automatically to let matter pass through from the small intestine into the colon, but closes automatically to prevent any substance, liquid or solid, from returning into or entering into the small intestine from the colon. If this happens, YOU'RE IN TROUBLE.

The ileo-cecal valve opens into the colon in a pouch known as the cecum which is somewhat larger than the other pouches constituting the colon. It is the first receptacle for waste residue.

The cecum does not always empty its contents into the colon immediately, and from this point onward we must, patiently and with tolerance, study this subject in some detail, whether we like it or not, as this region is one of the most vital areas controlling our indisposition, malady and infirmity on the one hand, or **VIBRANT HEALTH** on the other hand.

THIS IS AN OUTLINE OF THE DIGESTIVE SYSTEM

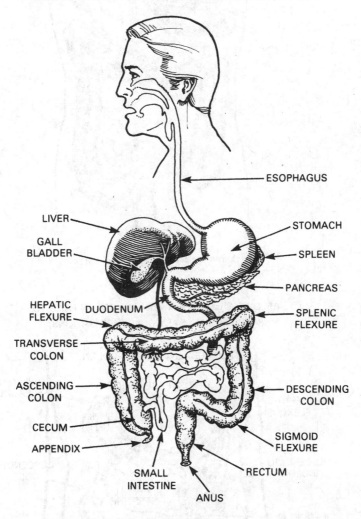

Food enters the mouth, goes down the esophagus and enters the stomach. The pyloric valve controls the passage of food from the stomach to the duodenum, where the bile and the pancreatic juices continue the processing.

From the duodenum the food travels through the small intestine from which liquefied nourishment goes to the liver. What cannot be digested is propelled to the ascending colon as waste. As debris and as feces for evacuation from the system.

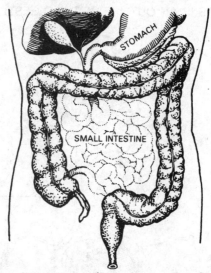

ABOVE: What a person's Colon should be.

BELOW: What happens when the COLON FAILS TO
RECEIVE NECESSARY COLON IRRIGATIONS.

BLOATED and SPASTIC COLON.

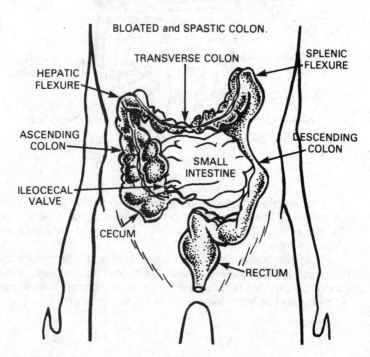

THIS IS THE ASCENDING COLON WITH SOLID IMPACTION OF FECAL MATTER, WITH ONLY A TINY HOLE, CLEAR IN THE CENTER.

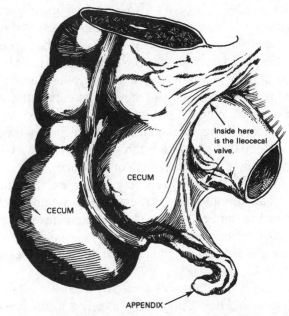

Inside here is the Ileocecal valve.

CECUM

CECUM

APPENDIX

THIS ILLUSTRATES THE LOWER PART OF THE ASCENDING COLON, SHOWING THE APPENDIX AND THE ILEOCEAL VALVE WITHIN THE JUNCTION OF THE SMALL INTESTINE WITH THE ASCENDING COLON.

The ileo - cecal valve is equipped with a safety mechanism which opens automatically to let matter pass through from the small intestine into the colon, but closes automatically to prevent any substance, liquid or solid from returning into or entering into the small intestine from the colon. If this happens, YOU'RE IN TROUBLE.

The ileo - cecal valve opens into the colon in a pouch known as the cecum which is somewhat larger than the other pouches constituting the colon. It is the first receptacle for waste residue.

The cecum does not always empty its contents into the colon immediately, and from this point onward we must, patiently and with tolerance, study this subject in some detail, whether we like it or not, as this region is one of the most vital areas controlling our indisposition, malady and infirmity on the one hand, or **VIBRANT HEALTH** on the other hand.

Chapter 11
GOOD MORNING!
HOW IS YOUR COLON THIS MORNING?

This is an excellent question for you to ask yourself, particularly when you wake up feeling groggy, heavy, dull, listless and negative. The chances are that waste matter in your colon has failed to be processed and expelled on schedule. This sluggishness is the beginning of a toxic condition which Nature is calling to your attention in order that you may remove the cause and prevent the cumulative effect of bacterial putrefaction before it becomes truly poisonous.

Headaches, undue weariness, fatigue are frequently the product of intestinal toxemia which spreads throughout the body. Cleansing the colon usually helps to correct such disturbances.

The cleansing of the colon is a very simple matter, although (I will admit) an awful nuisance. However, when we are working on such a vital and important project as the attainment of **VIBRANT HEALTH,** any interfering nuisance is simply waved aside. The goal is the ultimate and the most vital consideration, the achievement of **VIBRANT HEALTH.**

The cleansing of the colon is effected by means of enemas taken with a regular enema bag. This tube is attached to the rubber tube which comes with the enema bag and which is about four feet six inches in length. The details of how to take such an enema are given fully in my book **BECOME YOUNGER.**

The enema is the method suggested to go through the colon cleansing procedure at home.

There is a far more efficient cleansing process which is known as a Colon Irrigation, or a Colonic, or a Colon Lavage - all meaning exactly the same procedure. Such colonics are usually given by Physiotherapists, Chiropractors and Naturopathic Doctors. I am sure you will find one listed in the Yellow Pages of your Telephone Book under Colon Therapy or similar headings.

Experience has taught me that no health and healing procedures can be as successful as those which have a series of colon irrigations as the prelude to any health treatment. This makes sense, because just so long as there is material in the colon which may be conducive to the generation of poisons in the colon and to the diffusion of such poisons throughout the system, no healing can take place which is not the precursor of a chain reaction of ailments at a future date.

While it would be fanatical to dwell constantly and intensely on the condition of the colon, day in and day out, reason and intelligence will guide you to attend to your eliminative problems as and when necessary.

Colonics are, in effect, glorified enemas using many gallons of water - only an ounce or two at a time - and are given by the colonic operator, with the water flow and expulsion under the control of the operator, while the patient lies relaxed on the appropriate table connected with the colonic equipment. An efficient colon irrigation requires from three quarters of an hour to one hour, depending on the condition of the colon.

The prolonged retention of fecal matter in the colon may accumulate to such an extent that the walls of the colon may become thickly coated with such matter as you will see dramatically portrayed in the accompanying illustration. In this picture you will notice the colon has been cut across a section of it to show the thick impacted wall of the colon which has left only a tiny opening through the center for waste matter to pass through.

How The Colon Functions

The walls of the colon have an important function to perform, namely the squeezing of its contents to extract as much as possible of the liquid nourishment remaining in it, and pass this liquid by osmosis through the walls of the colon for diffusion throughout the body. A thickly impacted wall makes this function impossible of performance. The victim of such an impacted colon, may, under such conditions even have several "bowel movements daily without discomfort, but this condition is neither normal nor indicative of health! In fact it is an extremely dangerous situation as a complete blockage of the colon could take place at any time.

A Blocked Colon!

When a complete blockage of the colon has occurred, the surgeon's usual practice, in order to save the victim's life, is to perform a colostomy, the formation of an artificial anus by an opening into the colon from the outside of the skin. For the rest of the victim's life his feces evacuations take place through a tube into a bag hanging from his waist. Isn't it better to prevent this horrible procedure? Personally, I would prefer to die, rather than to subject myself to such an affliction.

Give some serious thought to this, and realize that my harping on this subject may be the means, some day, of saving your life, because you cannot live long with a completely blocked colon.

COLON THERAPY CHART

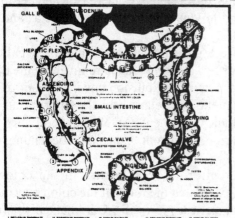

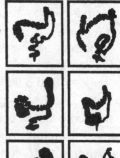

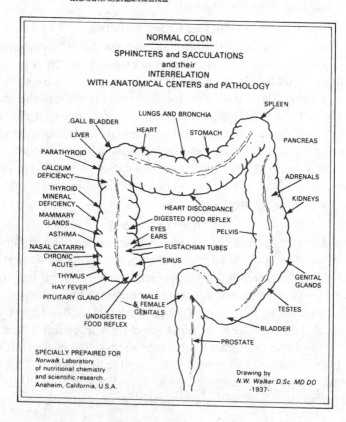

NORMAL COLON

SPHINCTERS and SACCULATIONS
and their
INTERRELATION
WITH ANATOMICAL CENTERS and PATHOLOGY

SPLEEN

LUNGS AND BRONCHIA

GALL BLADDER

HEART

STOMACH

LIVER

PANCREAS

PARATHYROID

CALCIUM
DEFICIENCY

ADRENALS

THYROID
MINERAL
DEFICIENCY

KIDNEYS

MAMMARY
GLANDS

HEART DISCORDANCE

DIGESTED FOOD REFLEX

ASTHMA

EYES
EARS

PELVIS

NASAL CATARRH

EUSTACHIAN TUBES

CHRONIC
ACUTE

SINUS

THYMUS

GENITAL
GLANDS

HAY FEVER

PITUITARY GLAND

MALE
& FEMALE
GENITALS

TESTES

UNDIGESTED
FOOD REFLEX

BLADDER

PROSTATE

SPECIALLY PREPARED FOR
Norwalk Laboratory
of nutritional chemistry
and scientific research.
Anaheim, California, U.S.A.

Drawing by
N.W. Walker D.Sc. MD DO
-1937-

BADLY IMPACTED COLON

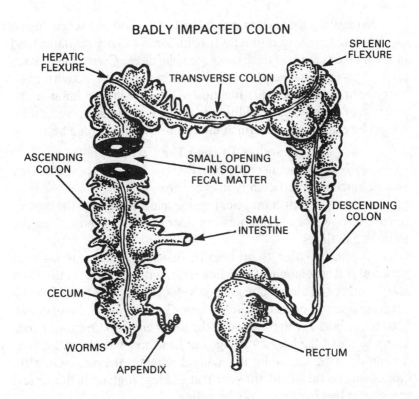

VIBRANT HEALTH compels you to be aware, alert and adamant in the proper elimination of waste products from your body without the use of drugs, laxatives or cathartics.

There is no laxative or cathartic which is not eventually harmful, at least to some degree. There is no cure for constipation by means of laxatives, as these merely serve to irritate the lining of the intestines and by such irritation the intestines try to expel the laxative medium, thus taking along some of the waste matter. The irritation to the intestines may eventually become the more serious problem.

The cleansing of the colon by the injection of water is a perfectly natural procedure. I have seen herons and egrets in the Everglades of Florida take water from rivers and streams into their long beak, insert their beak into their rectum, and have seen the water come out expelling masses of fecal matter. The rivers in India abound nearly all the time with birds going through that colonic procedure at the rivers' edge.

To keep the waste matter moving out of the body on schedule and the colon functioning normally it is important that your daily food intake include plenty of fresh raw vegetable juices. Carrot and spinach juice is particularly helpful in stimulating peristaltic activity. The beet juice mixtures help the function of the liver in its relation to the function of the colon. In addition to these, raw fruits and vegetables should be eaten daily to furnish the colon with the needed bulk.

Exercises To Help The Colon

A reasonable amount of physical exercise is vital to keep the body fit and functioning efficiently in every area.

Gardening, riding a bicycle, jogging and walking are the best all round exercises for out of doors. In-door exercises can be along the following outlines:

Using the regular "slant-board", or using a piece of 3/4 inch plywood 6 feet long and 16 inches wide, with one end on the floor and the other end elevated resting on a stool about 14 inches high and covering it with a piece of canvas, "monk's cloth" or similar material. Lie on this board with the head at the lower end, holding your hands on each side of the board; raising your head and body from the hips, up and down again, doing this daily a number of times. Or, also, while lying on the board, lift your feet and legs high up in the air and move your feet in circles, like bicycling.

Or, lie flat on the floor, raising your feet and legs from the hips, doing the windmill or bicycle exercise.

Or, put a pillow on the floor, kneel with your head on it and with your elbows touching the floor, raise your body up and down several times, keeping your knees, feet and hands on the floor.

Such exercises help not only to "tone up" the colon, but also the whole body.

Chapter 12
NUTRITION AND ENERGY; THE ENZYMES IN YOUR BODY AND IN YOUR FOOD.

The basic motive, reason and principle of Nutrition is to influence, induce and stimulate ENERGY. All other things being equal, energy is the sequel to proper nutrition.

Your body is composed of billions upon billions of cells which build the tissues constituting every part, organ and gland in your body.

Infinitely small as these cells in the body are, each individual cell is the composite of atomic elements, millions of such atoms being required for the structure of each individual cell.

Each individual atom is virtually a cosmic creation with a terrific volume of power within its core. This was clearly demonstrated in the splitting of the atom in the explosion of atomic bombs such as occurred at Hiroshima on August 6th 1945 and at Nagasaki, Japan, on August 9th of the same year. Even more powerful atom bombs have since been developed, using the hydrogen atom.

The atoms in your system are exactly the same as those which exploded those bombs. Don't get scared, though! Because no atoms in your system will ever explode in like manner, although the potential power and energy are nevertheless contained within them.

Just as your body is the composite structure of billions of atoms, so also is the atomic structure of all vegetables, fruits, nuts and seeds.

If you know anything about growing things in the garden you understand the importance of the care and nourishment which they require to grow and thrive. If they are neglected and do not receive their allotted care, food, and water, they wilt, wither and die. Your body is in exactly the same relative situation.

The cells in your body need nourishment to conform to the Law of Replenishment. This means that, as each cell furnishes you with its power and energy, it exhausts itself and must be replaced by a new one. The only means available to these cells to obtain their nourishment is by means of the food you eat and drink. If the cells in your body are well fed, and the exhausted and worn-out cells in addition to the residue of undigested substances are expelled from the body, there is every chance that **VIBRANT HEALTH** can be achieved and can be maintained, so long as this LIVE replenishment takes place.

Live Replenishment?
What Do I Mean By That?

By LIVE Replenishment I certainly do NOT mean that replenishment should take place by means of food which is swarming and alive with maggots!

I mean that fresh RAW food, vegetables, fruits, nuts and seeds are LIVE food because every atom composing them is imbued with the vital element we know as ENZYMES.

ENZYMES are not THINGS or SUBSTANCES. They are the LIFE PRINCIPLE in atoms and molecules. (Two or more atoms joined together form a molecule).

Consequently every cell in the structure of such vegetation is infused and animated with the silent LIFE known as ENZYMES.

Enzymes are as mysterious as LIFE itself. Enzymes are sensitive to all heat above 118° F, and at 130° F they are dead. Obviously any food which has been cooked at a temperature higher than 130° F has been subjected to the death sentence of its enzymes and is consequently dead food. Cold, even sub-zero freezing, on the other hand, does not affect enzymes.

Health, And Your Life-span.

Were it not for our Creator's foresight in regard to human weakness in the indulgence of one's appetites, humanity would have passed out of this world ages ago because of its existing mostly on cooked dead food. Howbeit, the human body has been invested with such a superabundance of both atoms and cells in its constitution, that it has been able to survive. Such survival, however, has been at the expense of a shorter and shorter life-span, and of an infinite number of ailments resulting from both malnutrition and failure to cleanse the system.

However, I am not satisfied with mere survival. I want **VIBRANT HEALTH** with its attendant vigor and energy.

Just as I am writing this paragraph, I am interrupted by a telephone call from a lady friend of ours who has only very recently been exposed to My Program. She was telephoning to say that last night she finally tried one of the salads detailed in my book **DIET & SALAD SUGGESTIONS,** which she and her family enjoyed tremendously. At midnight she decided to go further on My Program, and take a enema. She said she was astounded at the kind and quantity of waste matter which she eliminated by washing out her colon. This morning she felt so full of energy that she felt the impulse to telephone and tell us about it.

Nutrition and evacuation of waste from the body work hand in hand in building up the energy which is part and parcel of the VIBRANT HEALTH which gives strength, vigor and vitality. As I have clearly stated, both vegetation and the human body are composed of atomic elements. Both are live organisms whose atoms and cells are abundant with enzymes.

The enzymes in the cells of the human body are exactly like those in vegetation, and the atoms in the human body each has a corresponding affinity for like atoms which compose vegetation. Consequently, when certain atoms are needed to rebuild or replace body cells, there will come into play the magnetic attraction which will draw to such cells the exact kind and type of atomic elements needed for the work of replenishment or regeneration.

This magnetic affinity occurs in some mysterious manner in the liver as if the liver were a computer, and is directed by the functions of the Endocrine Glands.

Combinations of atoms constitute chemical structures whose efficiency is dependent on the enzymes in the atoms of the vegetable cells just as much as on the enzymes of the body. This constructive cell and enzyme work is what constitutes the assimilation of nourishment.

To understand this process is to appreciate the value of a raw food diet in relation to the attainment of health generally and of **VIBRANT HEALTH** in particular.

Chapter 13
CONSTRUCTIVE NUTRITION — OR DESTRUCTIVE FOODS; PART ONE: CARBOHYDRATES:

Sugars and Starches

Approximately 70% of the composition of your body is water. No nourishment can pass beyond the walls of the intestines and be taken into the system unless it has previously been processed by the digestive juices in the alimentary canal and converted into a liquid.

Only about 7% of all the elements composing your body is in the category of carbohydrates. Classified as chemical substances, carbohydrates are starches and sugars.

There is not one speck of starch in the composition of your whole body, nor can there be, because starch is not soluble in water and cannot therefore be converted into a liquid as a starch. Energy and exertion on the part of the digestive processes are required to convert the starches into sugars before the body can use them.

The carbohydrates in the composition of your body are in the form of sugars which are soluble in water and are consequently in liquid form which the body can use constructively. BUT the kind and type of sugar must be understood.

Chemically, sugars are divided into the following classifications, namely: cane, beet and corn sugars. These are manufactured products which are processed by intense heat and, being devoid of live enzymes, are consequently a hazard as food, and damaging to the human system.

The result of the conversion of starches into sugars by the digestive processes produces glucose or grape sugar in the body. Lactose, or milk-sugar, is present in the composition of milk.

It is necessary for you to understand these classifications and their purposes because "natural sugars" are present in the composition of all vegetation. Furthermore, the sweetening of food has become a necessity of more or less importance in order to make certain foods and their combinations more palatable.

Honey

Apart from all other facts and considerations, the body needs sugar, but it does NOT need the "refined" cane, corn or beet sugars. It needs, and can only use, "natural" sugars, constructively, the sugar present in raw vegetables and fruits and, best of all, HONEY.

The digestion of the commercial, industrial white sugar has a damaging, deleterious effect on the teeth, the gastrointestinal tract, the alimentary canal, and sometimes causing intestinal disorders such as diabetes, cancer, affliction of ones vision, pyorrhea, destroying the tissues of the gums, and loss of teeth. White sugar has a very destructive effect on women, increasing and intensifying pain during menstruation, aggravating nervousness and the weakness which, while generally considered "natural" is in fact utterly unnatural. Complete abstinence from white sugar, substituting honey in its place, has frequently prevented or stopped these discomforts.

To understand and comprehend the danger of using white sugar you must realize that food taken into the mouth takes from three to five hours to travel the 20 feet of small intestine. This sluggish, dawdling pace is necessary for the digestive processes in the intestine to disintegrate every particle of food you eat, and to liquefy it, in order that the atoms composing such food may pass by osmosis as a liquid through the walls of the intestine and, picked up by the blood, may be transported to the liver.

Incredibly, if the label on your honey container says "Uncooked", that honey has been heated. That is the legal term allowed processors who heat their honey up to 160°F for 30 minutes to kill the yeasts, retard granulation and to make it possible and easier to bottle the honey.

The vitamins, minerals and enzymes in LIVE unheated honey is what WE want.

Crystal clear honey has been heated and processed, deprived of its most essential vital elements, including the pollen.

It can be assumed that such heated honey has probably suffered some traumatic experience since the bees last saw it.

Sugar - Alcohol

White sugar does not have the patience to consume all that time to reach the liver. Actually, it becomes liquid before it has completed its passage through the stomach, then it fairly pours itself through the duodenum into the small intestine. By the time it has reached a little way into the small intestine it has been converted into alcohol and glucose. In this state it flows into the liver which is then swamped with an exorbitant volume of glucose. With the flooding of the liver with such glucose, the glucose is discharged into the blood causing an excessive amount of sugar to saturate the blood. The result is a blood-sugar affliction.

When the glucose content of the liver exceeds the point of tolerance the liver converts the glucose into fat globules.

Getting Fat

These fat globules are then discarded from the liver because their retention in the liver serves no useful purpose. What happens then? Just what people DON'T want to happen TO THEM! These fat globules are attracted to those muscles in the body which are more or less neglected in the person's exercises, namely the hips and over the stomach, besides being deposited under the chin.

Usually, on an average, it takes the first thirty years of one's life for these fat globules to change and enlarge the anatomical structure and contour of the victim of the sugar habit, and usually 30 to 40 years more before the fat is discarded - in the grave.

Let this be a warning to the younger generation. I consider white sugar a poison and I treat it as such. It has no place whatever in the program of **VIBRANT HEALTH.**

Refined and Fortified Starch

In regard to starches, as I have said, there is not a particle of starch in the constitution of your body. Starches, as such, are not soluble in water, and by starches I mean the cooked and processed grains, cereals and all processed flour products. They cannot be digested as starch.

Today bread and all starchy foods sold in the markets are made mostly from "refined" flour.

In people, refinement means elegance, loveliness, grace, neatness, and similar qualifications. In white flour the process of "refinement" has robbed the food of everything of constructive value, and not the least is the destruction of the enzymes. Nearly every vital element has been removed, eliminated or destroyed. To salve their conscience, the millers and manufacturers have added useless products and chemicals to "fortify" the flour and its products. "Refined" white flour is dead. I have never yet heard of a corpse being fortified to convert it into anything but a corpse.

It is impossible for man to improve on Nature by removing vital elements from foods and replacing them with manufactured products to fortify or reconstitute them.

White flour products, bread, cakes, crackers, and the like, are neither constructive nor regenerative. Therefore they have no place whatever in the achievement of **VIBRANT HEALTH.**

Fried Foods

Even more injurious is the use of fried flour products. When starchy foods are fried they are particularly pernicious. Why? Because, in the first place, the superheated fat is utterly UNdigestible. Then the fat-saturated starch cannot be effectively processed by the digestive juices, because of the conflict of interest, shall we say. It is virtually impossible for fat-saturated starch to be converted into any of the sugars. At the same time the fat which has been vitiated by excessive heat cannot be properly emulsified, and fats MUST be emulsified before the body can make use of them.

This deleterious combination results in the generation of unhealthy gas in the system, while giving a feeling of fullness and satisfaction for the time being. The end-product of the UNdigestion of foods cooked in fats or grease is putrefaction and fermentation of the residue by the time it reaches the colon, which can cause an offensive breath.

Malodorous gas and constipation are the natural sequence and the common result of eating such foods as donuts, fried potatoes, griddle cakes and the like.

In the beginning of this book I had in mind not quoting anything written by other authors, but I have in my library, in fact I have it here before me, a little publication which was printed some 127 years ago, which I think is particularly appropriate here. Besides, it is interesting to realize that people one and a quarter centuries ago were aware and conscious of the dangers of eating foods and drinking beverages which have a detrimental effect on the human system and which are neither useful nor conducive to the attainment of **VIBRANT HEALTH.** So, I will make a special chapter on DESTRUCTIVE FOODS which follows immediately.

Chapter 14
DESTRUCTIVE FOOD
DEVITALIZED WHITE FLOUR PRODUCTS:
WHITE BREAD, CRACKERS, DONUTS,
CAKES, ETC.

As I am typing this manuscript, I have before me a leaflet published by a Mr. Abel Haywood in England in 1845 - over 150 years ago. It covers the field of unwholesome foods "such as bread, cereals, etc." It reads as follows:

The title is:

An Inquiry Into The Cause Of Natural Death, Or Death From Old Age, Developing An Entirely New And Certain Method Of Preserving Active Healthy Life For An Extraordinary Period.

"Let it not be said that the life of man cannot be prolonged to many times the present period of his existence, because it is not so; as it was said that traveling by steam could never be accomplished, because passengers and luggage had been carried so long only by coaches and pack horses. It does not follow that because a thing is not, or has not been, that it therefore cannot be. Yet this is the common reasoning adopted by the world; this alone has been sufficient to bring ridicule, and even punishment and death, upon those who have ventured to propose anything out of the common path, even though it has ultimately been the source of great delight to the persecutors themselves.

"Human improvement, and progression, toward a better state of existence, will ever be retarded if discoveries and inventions are to be judged in such a foolish, unbecoming manner.

"Let the groundwork of every new subject be examined, and if found to be correct in principle - if truth be at the foundation - what has the world to fear from consequences?

"Are we so far wedded to old notions and practices, even though they constitute a very personification of falsehood and misery, that we are afraid of truth, and tremble lest it make us happier?

"The solid earthy matter which by gradual accumulation in the body brings on ossification, rigidity, decrepitude, and death, is principally phosphate of lime, or bone matter; carbonate of lime, or common chalk; and sulphate of lime, or plaster of Paris, with occasionally magnesia, and other earthy substances.

"We have seen that a process of consolidation begins at the earliest period of existence, and continues without interruption until the body is changed from a comparatively fluid, elastic and energetic state, to a solid, earthy, rigid, inactive condition which terminates in death. That infancy, childhood, youth, manhood, old age, decrepitude, are but so many different conditions of the body or stages of the process of consolidation and ossification - that the only difference in the body between old age and youth, is the greater density, toughness and rigidity, and the greater proportion of calcareous earthy matter which enters into its composition.

"The question now arises: what is the source of the calcareous earthy matter which thus accumulates in the system? It seems to be regarded as an axiom, that all the solids of the body are continually built up and renewed from the blood. If so, everything which these solids contain is derived from the blood; the solids contain phosphates and carbonate of lime which are therefore derived from the blood in which, as already shown, these earthy substances are invariably found to a greater or less extent.

"The blood is renewed from the chyle, which is always found upon analysis to contain the same earthy substances as the blood and the solids.

"The chyle is renewed from chyme, and ultimately from food and drink.

"The food and drink, then, which nourish the system, must, at the same time, be the primary source of the calcareous earthy matter which enters into the composition of the chyme, the chyle and the blood; and which is ultimately deposited in all the tissues, membranes, vessels, and solids of the body - producing old age, decrepitude and natural death.

"Bread, (from wheaten flour), when considered in reference to the amount of nutritious matter it contains, may with justice be called the staff of life; but in regard to earthy matter, we may with equal justice pronounce it the staff of death.

"Spring water contains an amount of earthy ingredients which is fearful to contemplate... It has been calculated that water of an average quality contains so much carbonate and other compounds of lime, that a person drinking an average quantity each day will, in 40 years, have taken as much into the body as would form a pillar of solid chalk or marble as large as a good sized man. So great is the amount of lime in spring water, that the quantity taken daily would alone be sufficient to choke up the system so as to bring on decrepitude and death long before we arrived at 20 years of age, were it not for the kidneys and other secreting organs throwing it off in considerable quantities.

"These organs, however, only discharge a portion of this matter; for instance, supposing ten parts to be taken during a day, 8 or 9 may be thrown out, and one or two lost somewhere in the body. This process continuing day after day and year after year, the solid matter at length accumulates, until the activity and flexibility of childhood becomes lost in the enfeebled rigidity of what is then called, though very erroneously, 'old age'.

"A familiar instance of earthy deposition and incrustation from water is observed in a common tea kettle or steam boiler. Every housewife knows that a vessel which is in constant use will soon become 'furred up', or plastered on the bottom and sides with a hard, stony substance. 4 and 5 pounds weight of this matter have been known to collect in 12 months. The reader must not mislead himself by thinking that because so much lime is found in a tea-kettle, the water after boiling is therefore free from lime. It is true, boiling water does cause a little carbonate of lime to precipitate, but the bulk of the sediment is left from that portion of the water only which is driven off by steam, or boiled away. This can easily be ascertained by testing the water both before and after boiling. It will be found to contain earthy particles however long the boiling may continue. Filtering it is also of no use, for this only removes what may be floating or mechanically mixed with the water, whereas the earthy matter here spoken of is held in solution. So that spring water, clear and transparent as it may appear, is nevertheless charged with a considerable amount of solid choking-up matter, and is, therefore, in any form unfit, or at least is not the best suited for internal use."

White Flour - The Staff of Death

Bear in mind that, at this writing, the foregoing was written and pulished some 150 years ago.

In his denunciation of bread as "the staff of death" Mr. Abel Haywood did not go into details sufficiently to clarify the reason for the impairment and damage which is caused to the human system by white bread.

Grains contain the largest concentration of starches, and that is where the problem lies. Up to 160 years or so ago, there was no such thing as the "white flour" of today. All flour coming from the flour mills was plain "whole" flour, with all its inherent natural nutritional elements retained.

Hungary, the foremost flour producing country in Europe, began using machines equipped with rollers to crush the grain, breaking down the cell structure. Further development resulted in the production of fine white flour followed by the Viennese bakers specializing in what became known then, and is still known today as, Vienna Rolls. As usual, Americans were quick to capitalize on the European fad for the Vienna Rolls specialty and the year 1880, or thereabouts, saw the Minnesota wheat industry embark in the production of white flour which, year after year, became more and more devitalized.

What a paradox and what an anomaly that for 4,000 years people used WHOLE GRAIN and when civilization entered a so called period of progress and enlightenment, nearly every vestige of life was taken out of grains when making flour!

One of the foremost exposers of the danger which faced civilization in the use of devitalized white flour was Sylvester Graham the great temperance and pure food advocate, born in 1794 and died in 1851. He advocated the use of the whole grain, unbolted and coarsely ground in making bread and other baked products. His specialty, Graham Bread, is still being produced and used to this day.

It is amazing to read syndicated stories by doctors proclaiming the virtues of "refined" white flour products and declaring them nutritious, in the face of all proof to the contrary. In fact, when the refining of flour first came into vogue, both in Europe and in the United States of America, foremost, prominent physicians remonstrated, denounced and condemned the practice of devitalizing flour as a step towards the deterioration of the health of the people. How far-seeing they were, and how true this has turned out to be.

The outer coatings of grains are composed of some of the most essential vitamins for the maintenance of health, such as biotin, riboflavin, nicotinic acid, to name a few. Without these, malnutrition results and ailments, such as constipation and many others follow suit.

Here are a few of the ailments which have sometimes been attributed to eating excessive amounts of devitalized flour products: dilation of the heart, acute anemia, swollen legs, paralysis.

Words are inadequate to express the danger of the consumption of baked foods made from devitalized white flour. Such food has no place whatever in the diet of ANYONE who aims to attain **VIBRANT HEALTH.**

From the financial, economic standpoint, it is better and cheaper by about 50% to buy dependable whole grains, grind them fresh as you use them, baking your own bread and other products, if you particularly want them.

Never overlook the fact that baking requires several times more heat than that of 130°F which is sufficient to destroy the enzymes. Nevertheless, there are people who think they need some bread and if they will limit their yearning to stone ground whole wheat or rye bread, and not more than one or two slices at a meal, occasionally, it may not do very much harm. But some raw vegetable or non-acid fruit should be eaten during the meal, even if it is simply one or two stalks of celery or some similar vegetable.

Whole grains need not be cooked. They can be soaked in hot water (125°F) overnight never letting the water come to a boil. When sufficiently soft they can be masticated comfortably, they are nutritious, and can be sweetened with honey, but they should never be sweetened with sugar. Eating some sprouted seeds with them is truly good and beneficial.

Chapter 15
CONSTRUCTIVE NUTRITION —
OR DESTRUCTIVE FOODS;
PART TWO: PROTEINS

How much protein do you need each day?

An infant requires a great deal more protein during the first and second years of life, in proportion to weight, than does an adult. The relative use of "protein building blocks" in the infant is greater because the body of the child is in the process of growing and developing.

An adult does not need, relatively, as much protein in proportion to weight, as a child does. The body of the adult needs no protein building blocks for structural building purposes. The adult needs protein only as repair blocks. The protein requirement of the adult is more constant and is limited chiefly to maintenance and replacement.

A person engaged in heavy muscular labor needs more protein than the individual engaged in sedentary work. This is why the person doing heavy labor usually eats larger meals. A person doing heavy labor needs at most 7 to 8 ounces of protein a day, while the sedentary worker needs no more than 4 ounces, although usually 2 ounces is sufficient.

Of course the kind and quality of protein is the determining factor. Do not overlook the fact that most of our protein intake is in the nitrogen which we breathe constantly. Nitrogen is the basic element in the structure of the protein molecule.

If the food eaten is easily digested and readily assimilated, then the amount of protein needed can be calculated at its minimum, say 4 to 6 ounces for the one doing heavy labor and 1½ to 2 ounces for the sedentary worker.

An important contributing factor in determining a person's protein requirement is the health of the individual. A loss of body tissue takes place in many diseases. This loss must be replaced during convalescence.

During and following such diseases the digestive system is naturally weakened. The nature of the protein is then a matter of grave importance.

All flesh foods require more exertion by the digestive processes than is the case with the digestion of vegetables. The digestion of flesh foods results in the generation of excessive amounts of uric acid. That being the case, feeding flesh foods to an invalid places an unduly heavy burden on the digestive processes while at the same time increasing the harmful acidity of the system.

The most constructive protein is available in the fresh raw vegetable juices. The combination of carrot-celery-parsley-and-spinach juices, classified as "potassium juice", is one of the richest sources of protein in the easily digested and assimilated vegetable juices category.

The juices of Brussels sprouts, savory cabbage, collards, dandelion, kohlrabi, lambs lettuce, parsley, salsify, spinach, turnips, all have individually relatively very high protein content. Such juices should always be taken with some carrot juice in their combination.

Garlic has the highest concentration of protein among the vegetables.

What Are Proteins?

Proteins are the building blocks of the human body and of all organisms. They are analogous to the bricks and cement blocks which constitute the structure of a building.

Protein is an organic substance characteristic of living matter present in various forms in the human body, and equally so in the bodies of animals and in plants.

The composition of proteins consists of some 23 microscopic substances known as amino acids. Each one of these amino acids performs functions characteristic of its particular activity. The best analogy I know is to compare these amino acids to all the functions and activities that go on day and night in office buildings of the sky-scraper type. In such buildings nearly every conceivable trade and profession is required to accomplish its operation and maintenance, from the lowest sub-basement to its flagpole on the roof.

So it is with the amino acids in your body. For example, one is a factor in the balance and operation of the adrenal glands, and in the condition of the skin and hair. Another is involved in the contraction of the muscles as well as in the structure and function of the reproductive organs, the control of the degeneration of body cells, etc. Another one is involved in the functions of the lungs and in the activities of the heart and of the blood vessels.

And so on, each amino acid has wonders to perform and I have listed these in my book **DIET & SALAD SUGGESTIONS.**

The interesting and vitally important thing about protein is that no *complete protein,* as such, can be digested and assimilated in the human system as a *complete* protein, whether it is animal flesh or other, irrespective of the number of amino acids composing it.

The colloidal or liquid amino acid atoms are transported to the liver by osmosis by the blood in the hepatic vein connecting the small intestine to the liver. It is the function of the liver to segregate and reclassify the atomic elements and re-combine them into the kind and type of amino acids and proteins required by the cells and tissues of the body, for the regeneration or replacement of such cells, for **VIBRANT HEALTH.**

The liver completely disregards and does not follow the advice or prescription of the manufacturer or dispenser of "protein products" as to the final disposition of such protein products. The liver is not educated to read "instructions", whether these are oral or in print on manufactured protein products.

Digestion Marches On!

The digestion of food actually begins when the vision or aroma of food alerts the Endocrine Glands to the fact that the functions and activities of the digestive juices are imminently needed.

As food is anticipated and it catches the eye, the visual and olfactory senses, the eyes and the nose, by the exercise of their role or business, stimulate the Endocrine Glands into activating the digestive organs, starting with the secretion of the parotid and other salivary glands in the mouth.

Mastication and chewing is a very important operation, because all solid food MUST be disintegrated and broken down into a mulch, and our teeth were given to us for that purpose.

Between the mastication by the teeth and mixing of the saliva, the food becomes a bolus known as chyme, a more or less rounded mass of broken-up food saturated with the saliva, ready for swallowing.

When swallowed, the chyme is propelled through the esophagus into the stomach. The glands in the stomach have, by that time, already been activated to secrete hydrochloric acid for the purpose of disinfecting whatever material is contained in the chyme, thus enabling the chyme to enter into a bath of hydrochloric acid.

Here is something worthy of note. Carbohydrate foods need an alkaline digestive medium for proper and complete processing, but they must first be disinfected in this hydrochloric acid bath, because the delicate lining of the intestine can be harmed or injured by the presence of infectious elements, besides the interference of such infection in the activity of the alkaline digestive juices.

Proteins, on the other hand, require an acid medium for the digestive juices to process them. Thus, when proteins enter the stomach and are being disinfected by the hydrochloric acid, the protein digestive juice pepsin is secreted by the glands in the stomach and the breaking down of the protein begins to take place.

Detrimental Chemical Reactions

When concentrated carbohydrates and proteins are eaten together, the carbohydrates are not properly digested if infiltrated by the acid pepsin protein-digestive juice.

Likewise, protein digestion is interfered with by the presence of the carbohydrates in the chyme. The result of these incompatible conditions is the fermentation of the carbohydrates and the putrefaction of the proteins. It is inevitable, due to natural chemical laws, that such an incompatible combination of fermentation and putrefaction should cause the generation of gas, not only in the stomach, but in the intestines and throughout the entire system.

In the program relating to **VIBRANT HEALTH** we try to rigidly avoid eating concentrated sugar and starchy foods during the same meal in which concentrated proteins are used, thus avoiding upset stomach, headaches, etc.

In chemistry, oil and water do not mix, nor do acids mix with alkaline substances. They are incompatible.

Carbohydrates are alkaline substances while proteins are acid. Carbohydrates are provided with their own specific digestive juices which operate in alkaline media and on alkaline substances. Likewise proteins are provided with their own specific digestive juices which process acid substances in an acid medium.

The natural sequence of this acid-alkaline chemical law is that trying to combine acid substances in alkaline media or trying to combine alkaline foods in acid media results in incompatible combinations causing a disruption of the digestive processes.

The outcome of this disruption is frequently the contributing factor in the vast majority of ailments, sickness and disease. The end product of the indigestion of incompatible combination of foods is fermentation and putrefaction, the basic elements of toxemia.

We have a definite line of demarcation between the Natural carbohydrates and proteins, and the concentrated. The Natural carbohydrates and proteins are the starches and sugars and the amino acids and proteins constituting vegetables, fruits, nuts and seeds in their natural state. In this constitution there is a relatively higher natural water content than there is in the flour carbohydrates, processed sugars and in the protein content of flesh foods.

Thus, all products made with flour, such as breads, cakes, crackers, spaghetti and other paste foods, are classified as *concentrated starches.* Candies and foods concocted from sugar, molasses, maple syrup, sorghum and the like are also classified as concentrated carbohydrates.

All flesh foods, beef, lamb, chicken, fish and products made to simulate these, and concocted from the protein of grains and legumes such as soy beans, etc., are classified as concentrated protein.

All Vegetables and Fruits Contain Protein and Carbohydrates

It is an easy matter to remember the difference between the Natural and the concentrated foods if we bear in mind that all vegetation contains both carbohydrates (in the form of Natural sugars) and proteins in the form best suited for processing by the human digestion, whereas the concentrated carbohydrates and proteins require a greater amount of digestive processing, thus causing more work and a greater burden on the digestive organs and their labor.

Some examples of food combinations to avoid being eaten together, are: Bread with eggs and flesh foods of any kind, coffee and sugar; Bread or bun sandwich with egg or meat of any kind, particularly when drinking "soft drinks", coffee or tea; Meat and potatoes with bread or biscuits, pie or cake, coffee, tea or "soft drinks".

Also soups containing flour or paste of any kind with meat stock or pieces of meat.

The more insidious harm is the eating of meat substitutes, because the protein-digestive juices are alerted to care for concentrated proteins, as the mind enjoys vicariously the flavor of meat. There being no protein present, these protein-digestive juices attack the "substitute" which is usually compounded from grains, or soy beans, and starches. The result is the INdigestibility of the food with repercussions of toxemia as the end product. These foods have no place in the diet for **VIBRANT HEALTH.**

Uric Acid

The basic reason for not eating meat, or at least for eating it sparingly if one considers it essential for the balance of his system, is the excessive amount of uric acid which is generated in the process of the digestion of meat and other concentrated proteins.

Uric acid is formed in the body naturally as a result of the activity of the muscles. Increased muscular activity is followed within an hour or two by an increased generation of uric acid which is excreted in the normal course of events through the urine.

During the processes by which flesh proteins are digested, resulting in the breaking down of the protein into its component amino acids, a certain amount of heat is liberated within the body which makes one feel stimulated and energetic. This helps to keep the body temperature up but it is not utilized for the energy needs of the working cells of the body. This amount of energy is therefore wasted and more protein would be needed than would be the case if all its potential energy were utilized. Therefore the amino acids from the meat thus ingested are not reconstructed into body protein and are virtually wasted, resulting in this uric acid being added to the uric acid resulting from muscular functions.

Uric acid is excreted through the kidneys, and most people who are large and frequent meat eaters are those most afflicted with kidney troubles. The presence of too much uric acid in the urine places a dangerous burden on the kidneys.

One of Nature's methods of warming up the body is to burn up its garbage into soluble ash which can be readily washed out of the body. This ash is known as urea which is so soluble that it never forms sand or gravel. If, however, there is excessive uric acid in the system, the body's fuel is not perfectly consumed and it forms an ash or clinker which cannot be washed out. This clinker is the uric acid forming into stones or gravel in the kidneys.

While stones in the gall bladder result from the excessive eating of concentrated starch foods, such foods can also cause the formation of stones in the kidneys.

Another danger of building up too great a supply of uric acid in the system, is its affinity for muscular tissues. Besides generating uric acid in their activities, muscles readily absorb and retain excessive uric acid when the kidneys become overloaded. The eventual result is the crystallizing of the uric acid into tiny sharp crystals which become very painfully manifest in rheumatism, neuritis and other muscular painful ailments.

Cease using meat and the aggravation may abate. Many people have found that drinking daily a pint or two of the juice combination of fresh raw carrots, beets, and cucumbers has helped to dissolve the excessive volume of uric acid crystals. In fact, this combination of juices has been found to be beneficial in helping relieve both liver and kidney discomforts. This information is given in much detail in my book **FRESH VEGETABLE AND FRUIT JUICES.**

When an individual actually feels he requires some flesh protein, then, it has been found, fresh fish which has fins and scales, has been used with benefit if the cooking has been limited to a matter of 10 or 15 minutes of steaming, but not frying it in fat or grease. Sea fish is preferable if fresh because sea food is the most complete of all foods, and sea fish contains virtually all the trace elements contained in the oceans. River and lake fish of the same characteristics - with fins and scales - are compatible because lakes and rivers also contain much of the elements washed into them from mountains, hills and valleys.

Bear in mind, however, that PERMISSIBLE is not the same as TOTAL ABSTINENCE!

Chapter 16
CONSTRUCTIVE NUTRITION —
OR DESTRUCTIVE FOODS;
PART THREE: FATS, OILS AND GREASE

Fats are a necessary requirement for the balanced maintenance of the functions and activities of the body.

Chemically, fats are a combination of glycerin and one or more fatty acids. Fatty acids are composed of the atomic elements carbon, hydrogen and oxygen.

Fats are divided into three classes: (1) Thin oils, such as vegetable oils: Sunflower seed oil, Sesame seed oil, Rice bran oil, Safflower oil, Walnut oil and Olive oil to name the principal ones. (2) Thick or heavy oils such as animal fats, and (3) grease, such as Crisco and other "shortenings".

For energy value, fats furnish 125% more energy than either carbohydrates (sugars) or proteins. Fats are also invaluable for maintaining the vitamin balance in the body as they are important carriers of Vitamins A, D, E and K, particularly, as these are all soluble in fat. A well balanced diet should take this into consideration and include the right kind of fats as important sources of these Vitamins.

Fats are essential components of cells and tissues of the body, BUT ONLY when the fats are natural fats which have not been subjected to excessive heat.

The digestive processes for the assimilation of fats require that fats be emulsified. Overheated fats cannot be so emulsified. Consequently such overheated fats, as well as any foods or food products which have been saturated by such overheated fats, cannot be properly digested. The result is not only the loss of the nutritional value of the food and the fat, but more serious is the end product of the passage of such fatty food through the small intestine being ejected from the small intestine into the colon to clog it up.

On the other hand, the unheated and unprocessed fats in all-raw salads, for example, are quickly and completely emulsified and oxidized when digested and assimilated by the body.

One of the functions of fats is to lubricate the joints in the bone structure of the body. With the phenomenal increase in the consumption of foods cooked in hot oil and grease, there has been a corresponding and alarming increase in the number of people having trouble and pain in their joints, such as bursitis, for example. Bursitis is inflammation of the joint caused by the drying up of the lubricant known as sinovial fluid which is secreted into the joints to keep them supple and free.

Untold millions of donuts, tons of fried chopped up meat known as hamburgers, pancakes, hot cakes and flap-jacks cooked on greased griddles, poultry fried in deep fat, just to name a few of the contributing factors causing the cumulative rise in creaking, painful, agonizing bones and joints whose sinovial lubrication has been deprived of its natural fat requirements. **VIBRANT HEALTH** shies away from foods cooked in overheated fats and oils.

Constipation is another corollary of eating foods cooked in excessively heated fats and oils, which are frequently heated over and over again. Natural fats are needed to act as lubricants to the intestinal tract in particular and to the entire body in general. A person whose body is deficient in lubricating fat has great difficulty in expelling feces and waste from the body.

The atomic elements iron and sodium are among the elements necessary to enable the blood to use sufficient oxygen for the complete combustion of the carbon composing the fatty acids. Failure to accomplish such combustion results in the accumulation of excessive amounts of fatty tissues - adipose tissues - usually where they are least wanted or desirable! Such a condition also affects the digestion and assimilation of proteins and carbohydrates which are then also diverted into the formation of adipose tissue.

Cold pressed oils are the only oils which are definitely beneficial and constructive.

The Laws of Chemistry apply to our food no less than to our digestive processes.

In order for fats to be digested they must be split up into glycerin and into the salts or atomic elements of the fatty acids. The presence of the atomic element sodium or other free alkaline atomic elements which are supplied by the bile and the pancreatic digestive juices are necessary for the splitting up processes of fatty acids known as emulsification. After being thus emulsified the product is transferred to the liver for absorption and reconversion into neutral fats.

Lard, margarine and fats, oils and greases which have been subjected to very high temperatures in order to process them have had their constructive nutritional value destroyed, any advertising propaganda to the contrary.

Avocados are the very finest source of fat that we can put into our body. All nuts contain good and a plentiful volume of fats, while all vegetables are imbued with fats in varying degrees.

Fried Foods Starve Your Body

If you eat fried foods you make it impossible for your digestion to completely nourish your body constructively because the overheated fat interferes with the function of the liver in the proper use of the atomic and molecular elements in your food.

The temperature of oils and fats used for cooking food varies from 350° F to 450° F. Olive oil, for instance, when used to fry food is readily heated to about 350° F at which temperature it decomposes. It is the same with similar oils.

Once you know that excessive heat completely destroys the value of any fat for nutritional purposes, you may want to do what we do, and that is, to diligently and assiduously avoid eating any food which has been fried.

Margarine Is Indigestible

This brings us to the question of using butter substitutes, such as margarine or oleomargarine. The claim is made that, being a vegetable product, oleomargarine should be preferred to butter, which is an animal product. The fact of the matter is that in the manufacture of margarine not only are very high temperatures used which prevent the use by the body of fat-soluble Vitamins, but chemicals, coloring matter and other ingredients are added which I certainly would not want to put into my system if I expect to retain my **VIBRANT HEALTH!**

Fats are divided into saturated and unsaturated fats; oils extracted cold pressed from vegetables and seeds are the unsaturated fats and are consequently low in cholesterol. All animal fats contain cholesterol as they are composed mostly of the saturated or heavier or thick fats.

Chapter 17
CHOLESTEROL:
FATS CONTINUED

Cholesterol is the unnecessary nightmare of far too many people who are fearful that a mouthful of fat will cause the rapid degeneration of their blood vessels and what not. As a matter of fact, the body needs cholesterol.

In nutrition the proper selection and use of fats is very important, as there is a plentiful supply of foods with lower saturated fatty acids and a correspondingly higher quantity of unsaturated fatty acids. Furthermore, all foods contain both these fatty acids. All we have to do is to select the correct vegetables, fruits, seeds, nuts and oils, and avoid or reduce the use of animal food, heavy fats and greases, particularly the manufactured grease products.

When people feel they *want* to eat flesh foods, then let them concentrate mainly on poultry obtained from farmers whose poultry is not kept imprisoned in cages, and on fish with fins and scales, omitting scavenger fish and crustaceans.

For your guidance I am listing some of the foods in which the UNsaturated fatty acids considerably exceed the saturated fatty acid content.

The numbers after each item in the following list indicate how many times more the UNsaturated fatty acids are present than the saturated fatty acids. Thus, for example, Avocado has 3½ times more UNsaturated fatty acids than the saturated.

Avocado 3½	Almonds 11	Brazil Nuts 4
Black Walnuts 15	Chickpea 10	Corn Meal 7½
Eggs 2	English Walnuts 13	Filberts or
Hickory Nuts 11	Millet 2	(Hazel Nuts) 18
Oats 3½	Olive Oil 8	Olives 8
Pistachio 8½	Pumpkin Seed 4½	Pecans 12
Rice 4½	Safflower Oil 11	Sesame Seed 7½
Sunflower Oil 8	Whole Wheat 5	

With this information as your guide you can choose your food intelligently and avoid eating food containing an excess of the saturated fatty acids with their correspondent excessive cholesterol.

In the matter of cholesterol as in every other element individually involved in nutrition, bear in mind the *source* of the information praising and recommending the product.

In the final analysis realize that the body requires a certain amount of fats to enable the human mechanism to function smoothly. The body of a man weighing, say, between 125 and 130 pounds will contain about 12 to 14 pounds of fat if he is in a fairly healthy condition, while the body of a woman of similar weight will contain between 32 and 37 pounds of fat.

This fat is essential because it serves as a food reserve and forms the most efficient concentrated fuel both for maintaining the normal temperature of the body and to furnish energy for the power to carry on the functions and activities of our daily existence.

As a source of energy, the sugar-carbohydrate of honey, for example, furnishes energy quickly. While the energy supplied by fats is slower in manifesting, fats have double the energy potential of carbohydrates and consequently have the advantage of producing twice the volume of heat but "burn" more slowly. For this slower burning quality, fats are more suitable as a storage material and fuel reserve.

In the process of digestion, the pancreatic juice processes the fats present in the composition of the food, making them available for use, storage and distribution by the liver. However, if the fats have been heated in excess of 125°F, they and any food cooked in such overheated fat, fail to be adequately treated by the pancreatic digestive juices and will not be available for use by the liver. They are wasted.

Chapter 18
YOUR LIFE IS IN YOUR BLOOD;
TAKE GOOD CARE OF IT!

Your blood is your Life-stream.

Your blood is as good as the air you breathe, as good as what you drink, as good as what you eat. Could you have a more complete synopsis or summary of the composite of your constitution?

The most important and vital element which you can put into your body is AIR.

AIR is composed of approximately 79% nitrogen atoms and about 21% oxygen atoms.

Nitrogen and oxygen are by far the foremost, essential elements we need to keep the body and soul together.

Nitrogen is the basis of the amino acids composing the proteins constituting every cell and tissue in the body. Without its necessary supply of nitrogen the body would quickly disintegrate.

Although we ingest nitrogen with everything we eat, the nitrogen from the air is our most constant supply, since the nitrogen in food is only obtained as often as we eat food. Air nitrogen we inhale constantly.

Oxygen is an equally essential element in our nutrition, furnishing the blood with the means to give the body its needed heat to maintain its functioning normally. As the element of combustion, oxygen also is used in the system to burn up and consume used-up and dead cells and tissues.

We can exist, pursuing the even tenor of our ways, without solid or liquid food for days, sometimes for weeks, on end, without perishing, but we cannot continue to live in our physical body more than a matter of minutes, without air.

Nitrogen, in the air we breathe, is gathered from the lungs by the blood and delivered to the liver. It is used through the liver for the repair and regeneration of the proteins throughout the body to supplement the nitrogen present in the food we eat and in the beverages we drink. When we breathe impure and polluted air, the nitrogen which we inhale is diluted to the degree of the percentage of pollution in the air. Such poisoned nitrogen infiltrates and poisons the cells and tissues of the body.

The same condition applies to the oxygen in the air we breathe. The oxygen is a more consistent and tangible carrier of pollution because, while the nitrogen reaches the liver almost instantly after we inhale, and is processed there, the oxygen we inhale is carried by the blood throughout the system, from head to foot. Whatever pollution is present in the inhalation of the air, becomes a detrimental affliction, first, in the region of the brain. It encases the Endocrine Gland system in the brain area with the nature of the pollutant, preventing the Glands from performing their work at their highest peak of efficiency. The pollutants then infiltrate the rest of the system, because every drop of blood in the body travels throughout the system constantly. About 10,000 to 11,000 quarts of blood are pumped by the heart throughout the body every 24 hours. Bear in mind that the TOTAL BLOOD SUPPLY of the body is only about FIVE QUARTS!

Every drop of liquid we put into our system and every mouthful of food we eat is broken down into its atomic constituents in the small intestine, by the processes of digestion. Once the atomic elements have been liberated from the chyme and are able to pass by osmosis through the walls of the intestine, it is the blood that transports them, first to the liver through the hepatic vein, then from the liver through the heart for distribution throughout the body, as the liver may have dictated.

Thus the blood is the life-line between the food and its ultimate destination to nourish the cells and tissues of the body.

The oxygen which we inhale and which is then contained in the blood, combines with the atomic element carbon in the food we eat, to form carbon dioxide (or carbonic acid gas), which is mostly expelled when we exhale through our breathing cycles. Carbon dioxide is a gas which is heavier than air and is incapable of sustaining respiration. If one should find himself in an atmosphere low in oxygen and high in carbon dioxide, he would suffocate. If as little as 14% or 15% of carbon dioxide is present in the air we breathe, we would die.

Carbon is one of the principal ingredients in the composition of carbohydrates. The eating of excessive amounts of carbohydrate foods with a deficiency or absence of fresh raw vegetables in meals, more or less regularly, causes what is known as starch poisoning. This is the result of the vast amount of carbon dioxide generated from the combustion of the carbon atoms in the food by the oxygen in the blood, which is not completely eliminated..

The rate of the heart-beats is regulated by the volume of carbon dioxide present in the blood. As we set any muscles in motion they produce carbon dioxide. This carbon dioxide is picked up by the blood and within ten seconds after the carbon dioxide has left the muscles, it causes the heart to beat more rapidly. Consequently, because of the large volume of carbon in carbohydrates, the more carbohydrates one eats, the greater is the danger of developing heart trouble. Eating carbohydrates should always be accompanied by fresh raw vegetables.

Overweight - Too Fat IS Dangerous!

That over-weight lady sitting in her corner in the restaurant, gorging herself with cakes and pastries is building up heart trouble for herself with prodigious speed.

That chubby boy or girl which parents proudly display as the prototype of exuberant health, is stuffed with carbohydrates, and heading for any or all of the afflictions which accompany this condition of the body.

A clean, pure blood stream is the keynote to the achievement of **VIBRANT HEALTH.**

Your Lungs

Your lungs are composed of some 400 million infinitesimally small bunches of grape-like globules which collect the air you breathe and instantly pass it on to the blood vessels encircling them. At one and the same time these globules collect from the blood the carbon dioxide which the body must expel and which is eliminated when we exhale. Pollutants in the atmosphere have the tendency to clog up these microscopic air passages.

Your lungs are the very life-line of your blood and upon them depends the degree of success you have in your attempt to achieve **VIBRANT HEALTH!**

To breathe the air in a room filled with tobacco smoke results in the pollution of the lungs. By far the most dangerous element in that stale tobacco smoke is the carbon monoxide. Carbon monoxide is a molecule composed of one carbon atom with one oxygen atom, whereas carbon dioxide is the molecule of one carbon atom with two oxygen atoms. The carbon dioxide present in excessive volume, will not sustain respiration whereas carbon monoxide is more deadly; 50 parts of carbon monoxide in one million parts of air is the maximum of breathing tolerance without danger, but tobacco smoke which contains 75 to 90 parts per million carbon monoxide fills a room with atmosphere that will poison people.

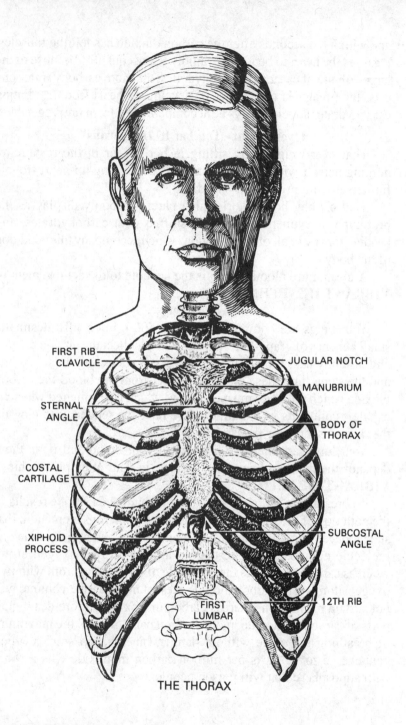

FIRST RIB
CLAVICLE

JUGULAR NOTCH

MANUBRIUM

STERNAL
ANGLE

BODY OF
THORAX

COSTAL
CARTILAGE

XIPHOID
PROCESS

SUBCOSTAL
ANGLE

12TH RIB

FIRST
LUMBAR

THE THORAX

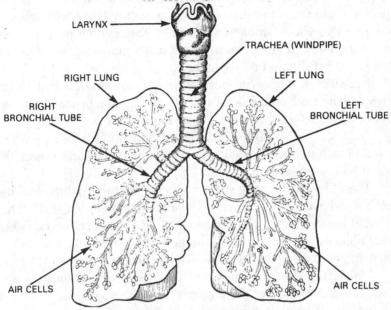

THE TRACHEA AND AIR-TUBES OF THE LUNGS

LARYNX

TRACHEA (WINDPIPE)

RIGHT LUNG

LEFT LUNG

RIGHT
BRONCHIAL TUBE

LEFT
BRONCHIAL TUBE

AIR CELLS

AIR CELLS

(Figure not accurate as to detail)

Your Life and Your Health at Stake -
Avoid Tobacco

Your blood is the most sensitive magnet in your body.

Tobacco smoke is an aerostatic gas which contains all the atomic elements emanating from the burning of tobacco.

Whether the smoker does or does not inhale the smoke while smoking makes little or no difference. Whatever smoke is in the mouth or in the nostrils pollutes the in-taking breath with the noxious gas of tobacco smoke.

A non-smoker in a room filled with tobacco smoke is subjected to the same toxic tobacco poisoning as is the one who is actually smoking.

This toxic poisoning is bad enough for a mature individual who chooses to exercise his inherent right of free-will as a free moral agent and smokes for cause or reason best known to him or to herself. It is a totally different matter, however, to subject others who detest or who are allergic to tobacco smoke, to have to breathe their polluted atmosphere.

After one of my lectures, some years ago, one of my students came to me and said:

"Dr. Walker, I have been working as accountant in a large firm in this City, and the entire premises are constantly filled with tobacco smoke. Everybody smokes, and I have been getting progressively more and more ill at ease at my work as I simply cannot stand that smoke. What should I do about it?"

I advised her to write out her resignation and hand it to the President himself, and if he asks for an explanation, just tell him your doctor advises you to work in a clean atmosphere.

"But, she said, I have been working in that office for 25 years!"

So much the better, I said. Just do as I suggest and I think the result will surprise you.

The following evening she came to me after my lecture, looking radiant and like a different person. I naturally thought she had left her job and found another. On the contrary. The President was shocked at reading her resignation, and immediately gave orders that from then on, there would be NO SMOKING permitted on the premises!

Unquestionably, the most insidious, repulsive, disgusting and disagreeable pollutant of the atmosphere is tobacco smoke. A smoker has no idea of how offensive tobacco smoke can be to a non-smoker.

Some people are under the illusion that cigar smoking is not as harmful as cigarette smoking and that it will not cause cancer. This is a false concept. Besides, the odor of cigar smoking is even more offensive than other tobacco smoke.

Tobacco has an evil insidious hold on people. Many have smoked until they developed cancer of the throat, underwent an operation, lost their power of speech, were rendered physically unable to smoke again, yet the intense desire for tobacco did not leave them, and constantly tormented them.

The insidious damage to a smoker's lungs and to his bloodstream, to his Endocrine Glands, to his cerebrospinal fluid, etc., makes no impression on his smokebefuddled cranium. The pollution of his blood with the concomitant effect of impairment on his health, mentality and longevity give him no concern.

Still more dangerous is the mother who smokes, exposing her offspring to the degeneration of its bloodstream and the undermining of its health. Furthermore, children are experts at mimicking, and seeing their parents smoke they consider it their prerogative to mimic and to emulate their elders.

It is truly shocking to find a non-smoking, wholesome, clean-living young man married to a woman who smokes constantly, notwithstanding the presence of their children.

I know a non-smoking fine young man who married a very lovely girl from a good family, not knowing that she smoked. They have two lovely children and, as frequently happens, she became a chain-smoker. A chain-smoking woman pollutes every room in the house and everything in it. There is no place at home to escape it. This young man loves his wife and children very dearly, so is very frustrated.

My father smoked, when I was a little boy. I figured it was alright for me to do what I saw him do every day. One day I stole some of his tobacco and made a cigarette with a piece of newspaper. I was quickly overcome by nausea "and the rest", and on top of all this I received a sound thrashing. This confused me because I thought perhaps I should not have used his tobacco, so I crushed some dried cabbage leaves and repeated the performance. So did he, when he discovered me. The results were similar - from the beginning to the end of my anatomy!

Now I should add that my father was a minister, a preacher, and a Baptist one at that. After that second thrashing I pondered long about the propriety of smoking being bad for me, an ignorant innocent child being spoon-fed religion, while it was permissible for a Minister of the Gospel to pollute his body with the same poison which caused me to vomit. To this day I cannot reconcile this anomaly!

Perhaps some day we will know the answer.

Chapter 19
BEVERAGES: GOOD AND BAD.

We MUST drink plenty of liquids in order to maintain the water-balance in our system.

The constitution of the human body consists of 65% to 70% water. About one gallon of water is eliminated from the body every 24 hours through the pores of the skin, through the kidneys and through other eliminative organs. In order to maintain the correct healthy waterbalance, this loss of water must be replenished.

About one gallon of the water in the body is a component of the blood and circulates under pressure by the pumping action of the heart. By means of this pressure the blood-water percolates through the tiny blood capillaries and permeates the space between the cells and tissues of the body, bathing in that water every cell in the system. This blood-water is known as lymph.

This constitutes the lymph circulating system. The lymph circulates throughout the body through its own circulatory channels. These channels are known as the lymphatic system.

The lymphatic system begins where the tissue fluids are first collected at the end of every blood vessel, through the network of lymph capillaries. The lymphatic vessels transport the lymph through the jugular vein into the heart for circulation. Here it drains from the right side of the chest, from the right arm, and from the right side of the head. All the rest of the body drains the lymph into the thoracic duct of the liver in the upper chest.

Beware Of Soft Drinks!

It is one of the functions of the lymph to collect toxic material out of the blood and from other parts of the body.

Let this become an indelible fact in your mind if you are interested in **VIBRANT HEALTH:**

Whatever you put into your mouth to eat or drink, goes into the blood first, then the lymph extracts the toxins. Furthermore, the lymph collects also noxious material and bacteria anywhere in your system to prevent their entering into the blood stream.

When the lymphatic system has reached the point of tolerance for toxic and noxious material, the lymph glands become engorged. The final product of such engorgement may be tumors, cancer, elephantiasis, Hodgkins disease, leukemia and other ailments in which such engorgement is a contributing factor. It is therefore very well worth while having **VIBRANT HEALTH** in mind when tempted to eat or drink what is not constructive nourishment for our system.

"Soft drinks do not belong in the healthy human system, much less in the sickly body. Do you have any idea of what enters into the manufacture of "soft drinks"? Sugar and carbon dioxide, to begin with. To drink it, you are adding additional carbon dioxide to the already superfluous volume of it in your body, thereby increasing your heart-beat and doing other damage of which you may not be currently aware, nor to connect eventual ailments to the cumulative damage done to your body by such drinks.

This carbon dioxide may have been extracted from the charcoal industry or by the reaction of chalk or bicarbonate of soda with sulfuric acid. Likewise, the "purest white sugar" is used to produce "soft drinks", sugar which, besides being deprived of every vestige of nutrition, is treated with excessive heat and with sulphuric acid. Phosphoric acid is another ingredient, and a corrosive one at that. The coloring matter which attracts the eye and deceives the mind are coal tar products which are harmful to the delicate digestive system.

Summing it up, it is my considered and conclusive judgment that such "soft drinks" help to destroy the body way ahead of its allotted life-span.

Beer Destroys Kidneys

Beer helps to degenerate the kidneys. Britons and Germans are drinkers of beer, ale and stout. Britain has among the highest rate of kidney degeneration among civilized countries except only Germany. The U.S.A. is fast catching up with these countries.

Alcohol is well known as one of man's most destructive physical, mental and spiritual assassins. Alcohol is the only substance that enters into the blood stream and into the human system through the walls of the stomach without necessarily going through the processes of digestion. It reaches the brain area almost instantly after it is swallowed and so affects the brain and the Endocrine Gland system.

Milk Produces Excess Mucus

Milk is not intended as a beverage, by Nature. It is the food for the infant, and meant only for the use of the kind from which it is derived. This is basic, although there are circumstances that do alter cases. Nevertheless, cow's milk is the most mucus-forming food in the human dietary. This subject is covered effectively in my books **FRESH VEGETABLE AND FRUIT JUICES** and **GUIDE TO DIET & SALAD.**

The truly constructive beverages are those which are replete with enzymes, and this condenses the choice to the fresh raw vegetable and fruit juices, and herb teas. There are thousands of different herbs available to man. These are both useful and constructive and their value is inestimable. They should not be boiled. Herbs should be steeped in hot water at a temperature of not much over 125°F in order to obtain the best benefit from them.

Bearing in mind all I have related in this chapter, THINK before you drink, and keep in mind the path which leads to **VIBRANT HEALTH!**

Chapter 20
YOUR ENDOCRINE GLANDS

Endocrine Glands are glands of internal secretion. That is to say, they secrete or generate hormones, which are extremely powerful elements used in ultramicroscopic amounts and injected by osmosis through the walls of the glands directly into the blood. These glands have no ducts or outlets.

The secretion of these hormones is most mysterious, yet the body would never be in balance or able to function properly without them. There is hardly an activity of the human body that does not in some way, directly or indirectly, require the use of hormones.

There is a constant action and inter-action between all the Endocrine Glands, and the instant manner in which they project their hormones even to the most distant parts of the body, is nothing short of miraculous. It staggers the imagination to try to figure out how a tiny drop of blood is impregnated with a hormone and in an instant deposits that hormone exactly where it is called for. Furthermore, when different kinds of hormones, be it a few or a dozen, are all called for at once, each one arrives at its destination immediately! Some to the head, some to the midriff, some to your toes, with never a delay or a mistake.

It is difficult for the mind to grasp the fact that the primary energy which enables the glands to function and operate is that elusive Cosmic Force which is the basis of life and activity in everything in this Universe.

The Pineal Gland is the antenna or receiving station of this Cosmic Energy or Force, which, upon entering the body, is condensed to a voltage which the individual body can tolerate and use, and it automatically infiltrates every Endocrine Gland and other organs and parts of the body. This is the mysterious, secret reason why you are able to keep body, soul and spirit together, and to function as you do, year in, year out, for scores of years.

This Cosmic Life Force is eternal and indestructible, it is only the anatomy which is subject to decay, degeneration and destruction, unless it is constantly replenished with the necessary elements to regenerate and revitalize the cells and tissues composing it.

Other elements, of course, also enter into this process of degeneration. We have already listed some of these. They are the negative emotions which can undermine the constitution of the human body and destroy it.

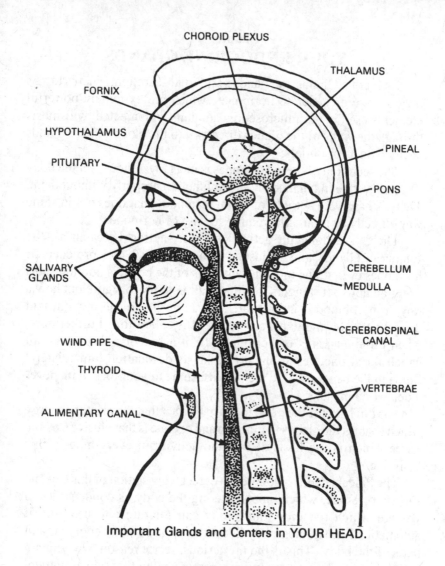

Important Glands and Centers in YOUR HEAD.

The following labels appear in the diagram:

CHOROID PLEXUS

THALAMUS

FORNIX

HYPOTHALAMUS

PINEAL

PITUITARY

PONS

CEREBELLUM

MEDULLA

SALIVARY GLANDS

CEREBROSPINAL CANAL

WIND PIPE

THYROID

VERTEBRAE

ALIMENTARY CANAL

The Liver

The Liver is the largest, the most complex, and one of the most constantly active endocrine glands in your system.

When you consider the vast number of ailments in which the liver is involved, directly, you will realize how important are its disfunctions resulting from man's lack of knowledge of body functions.

Some of the most commonly known ailments and discomforts resulting from liver trouble, are: constipation, diarrhea, hemorrhoids, gall stones, jaundice, biliousness, diabetes, depression, drowsiness, nausea, mental strain, abscesses, warts, sclerosis of the liver to name just a few.

With such a revealing list of calamities in mind, the desire for self preservation and the urge to attain VIBRANT HEALTH should lead every one reading these pages to become educated on how the body functions. Then take HEALTH seriously and begin training one's appetites and emotions with rigid discipline, omitting damaging and evil habits at all costs.

Metabolism

Metabolism involves the chemical changes in living cells by which the energy is provided for the vital processes and activities, and new material is assimilated to repair the waste.

Actually, metabolism involves the transformation and converting of nutritional elements in food-stuffs into simple principles in the regeneration of the cells and tissues of the body so that these can furnish us with the energy needed for our living processes.

Naturally, if metabolism is involved in live, organic nutritional elements of food the processes of conversion follow natural easy-flowing functions. If, however, the enzymes in the food have been destroyed by cooking with excessive heat, or with heat processing, there is no vitality in the food and the metabolism involved in their processing in the body labors under stress and with handicaps. It is under these circumstances that toxemia develops.

Food without live enzymes, could not respond to the requirements of metabolism without some compensating operations, in which case the molecules in the body area involved would have to overwork and many energy producing atoms involved in this overwork would fail to obtain replenishment or regeneration and would become expended. This condition can continue for years on end, but the day of reckoning arrives unexpectedly when deficiency ailments overtake the individual.

All food eaten must be liquefied by the digestive processes and the component atoms and molecules separated in order that they may pass by osmosis through the walls of the intestine for transportation to the liver by means of the portal vein.

It strains the imagination to try to imagine the millions upon millions of atoms separated from the fiber structure which composed the food, all mixed together in an apparent jumble, streaming through the infinitely small microscopic villi or tubes in the walls of the intestine before they can reach the liver.

This miraculous operation is possible because of the regulation and control exerted by the Endocrine Glands in every function and activity of the human system, particularly in metabolism. Each Gland, in its own sphere of activity, exerts its influence on the functions evolving within the cells of the liver.

The internal secretions of the liver work on the metabolism of carbohydrates, proteins and fats received from the small intestine and reconstructs into the components as required and called for by the body.

Liver Process of Starches and Sugars

Although food must pass through some 20 feet of small intestine before its nutritional elements can reach the liver, there is usually still some nourishment in the residue leaving the small intestine to enter the colon. While the function of the colon is to evacuate matter from which the small intestine has extracted nourishment, there nevertheless always remains some particles of nourishment in the residue. It is consequently the function of the first half of the colon to extricate from its contents whatever nourishing elements are present in it, transfer them by osmosis into the blood which in turn transports them to the liver.

You can well imagine the poisoned state of such elements when they mix with putrefied corrupt feces which has accumulated in the colon due to constipation and other evacuation delays!

What an amazingly wonderful body you have been entrusted with by your Creator!

Carbohydrates comprise the starches and the sugars. Starches, as such, would quickly clog up the system if allowed to enter the liver.

Starches are first processed in the mouth by the saliva. This is the first process of digestion to convert starches into sugars. Then by the digestive juices in the small intestine until the conversion into sugars is completed. Starch will not dissolve in water, but sugar does.

The liquefied sugar reaches the liver through the wall of the intestine and by the portal vein. Upon reaching the liver the glycogen is secreted, converting the sugar into glucose.

Glucose is stored in the cells of the liver until the body requirements call for sugar for heat and energy. The glycogen then re-converts the glucose into the type of sugar required by the cells and tissues in the body and injects it into the blood in the hepatic vein for transportation to its destination.

Do not overload the body with concentrated starches and sugars, if you want to enjoy **VIBRANT HEALTH.**

Liver Process of Proteins

Protein is an organic substance consisting essentially of the atomic elements carbon, hydrogen, nitrogen, oxygen. Protein is characteristic of living matter and found, in various forms, in humans, animals and plants.

Proteins are the main constituents of the cells and tissues of the body and are composed of about 23 varieties of amino acids. No protein, nor any of the amino acids enters the liver, as such, from the food ingested through the intestine.

All protein and amino acids of every kind and nature are broken down in the process of digestion through the alimentary canal, into the simple atoms and molecules composing them. These separated elements reach the liver as individual atoms and molecules. The processing by the liver must reassemble and re-convert these into such amino acids and proteins as are needed for the regeneration and replenishment of the used-up cells and tissues in the body.

There are three sources from which the liver receives material for the reconstruction of needed amino acids and protein, namely:

First: from the protein content of vegetables, fruits, nuts and seeds, and from fresh raw vegetable and fruit juices.

Second: from the concentrated protein of the flesh of animals, fish and fowl, and from the concentrated food "supplements"

Third.: from the air we breathe.

The first and second items are generally understood.

The third source, AIR, while familiar to every living creature, is not generally understood, considered and appreciated as necessary protein nourishment. The air we breathe is composed approximately of 80% nitrogen and 20% oxygen. Nitrogen is an essential constituent of all the amino acids and proteins.

The oxygen sustains respiration and constitutes an important percentage of organized human and animal bodies. Oxygen generates heat. All amino acids are composed of nitrogen, oxygen, hydrogen and carbon. The carbon composing our food is constantly consumed by the oxygen we breathe, which is collected and distributed throughout the anatomy by the blood.

The nitrogen which we breathe in the air is transported by the blood to the liver where it is converted into one of the atomic or molecular ingredients for the reconstruction of amino acids with which to build cell proteins.

It is false to claim that we MUST supply our body with "complete protein". What the body does need is the material, in the form of the right kind of atoms and molecules, with which it can build the type of protein called for by the cells and tissues of the body, to achieve **VIBRANT HEALTH.**

What Is A Complete Protein?

A "complete" protein would contain all of the 23 amino acids. It is a physical impossibility for the liver to receive a "complete protein", as such. Such protein must first be completely disintegrated into its component atoms and molecules by being processed through the alimentary canal.

If this is not quite clear to you, then stop and think: Would you eat a WHOLE live rooster, or grouse, or pheasant, or duck or goose? No, indeed, you would NOT! You would first separate its life activity from its body by cutting off its head. You would then pluck off all its feathers; next, you would process it by cleaning out its innards, then cutting it up into convenient sections for cooking and eating, and even then, when you eat it you would only eat one mouthful at a time. Right?

By analogy that is what happens to the proteins you eat. Every piece of flesh, animal, fish or fowl protein is composed of amino acids, and every amino acid is composed of atoms and molecules in certain definite amounts and proportions.

Your digestive system processes these proteins and amino acids so that their atoms and molecules can pass through the wall of the intestine to the liver where they are reassembled and reconverted into the type of protein needed by the cells and tissues of the body.

Each molecule must be disintegrated in the processing by the digestive system in order to reach the liver for reconstruction and distribution as nourishment for the cells and tissues of the body.

Liver Process of Fats

The quantity and the quality of the fats in our food and in our bodies seems to be a mystery to most people. This subject of Fat is the most prevalent paradox disturbing many humans. Fat people want to become thin while slim people want to "put on" weight. Such is human nature. How fats function as they do, in the system, and cause the end-result, is often unpredictable.

One person can fast for several days and instead of losing weight will find, to her dismay, that extra pounds have been added. On the other hand a slim person may eat enormous quantities of food and still add no weight.

Basically, fats are combinations of acids, the molecules of which consist of the atomic elements carbon, oxygen and hydrogen. It is the volume and the pattern or arrangement of each of these three elements in the molecules that cause fats to be thin oil, such as vegetable oils, or thick and solid, such as animal fats.

Like all other foods, no fats can be utilized by the body unless and until their molecules are broken down into their component atomic elements.

It is in the process of fat metabolism that fats are emulsified and reduced into their primary acid elements for collection into the liver, which then distributes them throughout the body.

Fats are formed by the combination of certain acids with glycerin, the acids being compounds of oxygen, carbon and hydrogen. When these elements get out of balance fat will be deposited as adipose tissue in those parts of the body where generally they are least desirable.

In childhood a certain amount of plumpness is tolerated if it is well distributed, and when it follows naturally if the child's diet is well balanced. However, too much fat in children predisposes them to enlarged tonsils, adenoids, and lymph glands. Also, such children are more inclined to develop excessive mucus resulting in colds and the usual "diseases of childhood".

After the adolescent stage has been passed, excessive fatness and disease are virtually synonymous. Fat people do not know what real health is and in the course of time are most likely to succumb to pneumonia, apoplexy, arteriosclerosis and other fatal ailments.

Upon reaching the mature age of the thirties, one's aim should be toward slimness. Such aim can be achieved by not overeating.

Exercise and the control of the kind and quantity of food eaten are essential steps to reduce overweight and retain slimness.

Posture is a habit very much generally neglected at this stage of life, and in later years. Yet careful attention to ones posture will help the toning up of the entire system as it keeps one constantly alert to the condition of the body.

To Lose Weight

Naturally, the very first procedure, when working on reducing one's weight, is the thorough cleansing of the colon by means of colon irrigations. This is natural and perfectly logical, because much of the adipose tissue is the result of the accumulation of waste in the intestines which prevented the proper assimilation of food and the complete elimination of waste residue.

Of course one must not overlook the fact that the emotions have a terrific bearing on the accumulation of excessive fat. Emotions have a powerful influence on the Endocrine Glands and CAN be controlled. If one controls one's emotions the Glands will cooperate and respond in kind. Failing to control the emotions disrupts the balance and equilibrium of Gland activity and causes a corresponding disruption in the metabolism of fats. The result is the deposit of fats as adipose tissue instead of burning them up as energy fuel.

The volume of food intake does not always result in overweight when eating excessive amounts of food. As a matter of fact many a thin person has grown thin because of eating so much more than necessary that the digestive and assimilative processes are overworked and become inefficient.

There is one secret and one key to the attainment of **VIBRANT HEALTH.** That is MODERATION in everything.

It is dangerous to take medicines to reduce, and just as dangerous to take medicines to put on weight. Apart from the fact that in principle such medicines are injurious and disrupt the body's metabolism, they do not attack the cause and at best they are no more than temporary remedies.

Fasting

Instead of taking medication in order either to reduce or to gain weight, it is wiser to undertake a controlled fasting program. *Under no circumstances should one fast for more than six or seven consecutive days.* The cleansing of the colon DAILY during a fast is essential to prevent the reabsorption of toxins during the period that the body is undergoing cleansing. If such a period of fasting is not sufficient, then similar periods can be repeated after intervals of at least three or four days.

Bear in mind that a prolonged fast exceeding 6 or 7 days will start a reversing process in the body. This means that the cells of the body will begin to feed on each other, lacking proper and natural nourishment. This could be very dangerous and may even become fatal.

During a fast, no solid food should be eaten, but at least one gallon a day of good pure water or diluted fresh raw fruit juices should be used as beverage, without fail. After a fast, no large quantities of solid food should be eaten for at least three or four days, as the body, having had the opportunity to rest from digestive labors and to relax, would rebel at so much sudden digestive activity. The best nourishment after a fast is the use of fresh raw vegetable juices together with a few fresh raw vegetables and some fresh raw fruits, for the following few days.

Do not be misled by the "Table of Weights" generally in vogue for people. No two people are alike and the structure and height and in fact the general build of the body should be the determining factor. You never see a race horse, in training, pulling a plow. Likewise, you never see a draft horse or a plow horse competing with race horses on the track. So it is with humans. Some people are overflowing with nervous tension and energy while others are equally phlegmatic. To achieve the proper balance and control between these is to come a long way towards achieving **VIBRANT HEALTH.**

When all is said and done, the liver carries the brunt of man's negligence in failing to eat the best possible kind and quality of nourishment. You are the one who suffers if the liver is unable to operate at its maximum level of efficiency. Energy is the most vital and essential element to maintain the body in proper balance and to enable one to live efficiently and more abundantly. When the body requires energy it obtains it from the oxidation of the fat stored in the liver.

Considering the material in the foregoing pages, you can appreciate the colossal amount of labor in which the liver is involved. When you assess the reorganizing of starches and sugars, the reassembling of the amino acids for protein, and the emulsifying of fats, is it any wonder that neglect to properly nourish the body results in liver ailments?

The liver is seriously affected by alcohol and nicotine, by excessive amounts of uric acid resulting from eating too much flesh foods too frequently, by food fried in oil, fat or grease, and by too much starch and sugar foods.

The most constructive special nourishment for the liver is obtained from honey, which it quickly converts into glycogen, and from the fresh juice of the combination of raw carrots, beets and cucumbers. These are the basic liver-food ingredients in **VIBRANT HEALTH.**

Chapter 21
YOUR HYPOTHALAMUS:

Your HYPOTHALAMUS is not exactly a Gland, but it certainly is involved in such a great diversity and number of functions and activities that every gland in your body is directly or indirectly influenced by it. It is one of the most vital and important focal centers of the human system.

An understanding of the ramifications of the workings of the hypothalamus could relieve the mind of many fears and frustrations. Properly attending to the many requirements of the body, and controlling the mind and the emotions will help to keep it in balance.

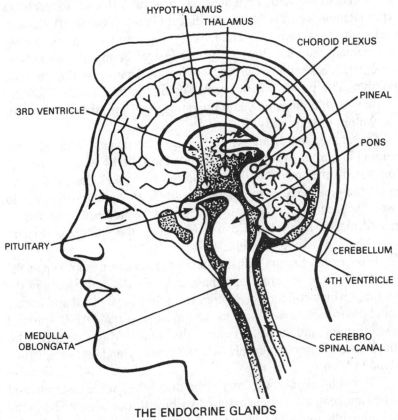

THE ENDOCRINE GLANDS

Actually, the Hypothalamus is a bundle of fibers and cells in the very center of the skull and the midbrain. Nearly every phenomenon in the operations of the Endocrine Glands involves the hypothalamus.

The eyes, the auditory system, metabolism, blood pressure (both high and low), water excretion, body-water balance, temperature regulation, appetite and hunger, sleepwalking phenomenon, in fact virtually every mental, physical and spiritual function and activity is in some way directly or indirectly influenced or controlled by the functions of the hypothalamus.

Fifty years ago the hypothalamus was just beginning to get recognition, but its vast field of activity has taken all the intervening time until now to just barely discover the high points of its value to our daily life.

Your Electric Life Force

To enable you to discern the first powerful influence to reach the hypothalamus we must study the Pineal Gland. The pineal gland is analogous to a radio antenna, receiving from the atmospheric environment the vital flow of Cosmic Energy acting like an electric current when it enters the body. Cosmic Energy is that infinite unfathomable power which permeates the entire Universe holding the planets in their course and operating right into the very core of every atom in your body.

Like the current from one of the huge electric generating stations sending hundreds of thousands of volts through the wires to the 115 volt transformer near your home, so the Universal Cosmic Energy enters the pineal gland with inexpressibly high voltage which would virtually burn up the body if the body were not equipped with a transformer to lower that Cosmic Energy to the voltage consistent with the needs of the individual.

The Cosmic Energy transformer in the midbrain is known as the THALAMUS, a structure of a mass of gray cells and tissues in the midbrain which collects the Energy from the pineal gland and lowers it and controls it to conform to the physical, mental AND spiritual development and needs of the individual. Many people who understand this procedure classify the pineal gland as the Spiritual Gland in Man.

The hypothalamus is located immediately below the thalamus and is the first center to collect and to distribute throughout the body the activating phenomenon of Cosmic Energy, generally spoken of as the Life Force.

The most vital fluid in the body is known as the cerebrospinal fluid. This fluid is charged with more of this energy, or life force, than any other part of the body except the pineal gland and the thalamus. The cerebrospinal fluid flows through the spinal column, fills the eye balls, lubricates the auditory system and bathes the inner core of every nerve in the body. Every gland in the body is dependent on the cerebrospinal fluid for its sensitive operation, and this includes the hypothalamus.

The hypothalamus is immediately above the Pituitary Gland, and by means of a network of nerves and blood vessels which pass through the pituitary, exerts influence or control over the functions and activities of the adrenal glands, the thyroid, the liver, the pancreas, the testes in the male and the ovaries in the female. The hormones secreted by these various glands are activated by the influence of the hypothalamus.

The kidneys are to a great extent regulated by the hormone producing influence of the hypothalamus through the pituitary gland. Many disturbances of the urinary functions emanate from a disturbance of the hypothalamus.

Emotional upsets have a direct bearing on the hypothalamus, affecting the blood pressure throughout the entire system and particularly in relation to the heart. To *know* this, means that every person who is "quick on the trigger" would do well to count ten before speaking or acting under such pressure while it exists, and give the blood circulation the opportunity to level off to normal.

Does Heat Or Cold Bother You?

The hypothalamus is truly your thermometer. Like any other part of your body, the hypothalamus is also subject to tumors or lesions when the body has been neglected in the matter of internal cleanliness and failure to eat sufficient raw foods, particularly when such foods are obtainable in the form of fresh raw vegetable juices. When a tumor or a lesion develops in the Hypothalamus, which is rare, it could cause the body to lose its ability to cope with changes in temperature.

When the body is properly cared for and the hypothalamus is in a healthy condition, the hypothalamus activates the necessary nerve mechanism to dissipate excessive heat by stimulating the respiratory and the heart pressure apparatus and the spinal cord. When the blood temperature has been raised to the necessary degree perspiration should begin, then the body temperature would automatically become normal and you are comfortable.

In cold conditions the hypothalamus influences the slowing down of heat evaporation from the system resulting in the body conserving heat.

Heat production in the body is also generated by the general speeding up of metabolism by the Hypothalamus. This function involves also the thyroid gland. All the blood which circulates through the body passes through the thyroid, consequently any noxious elements in the blood affect not only the thyroid but also the hypothalamus.

The presence of noxious substances in the blood stream which reach the hypothalamus usually result in affecting this valuable thermostatic equipment causing a disruption in its normal operation. Such noxious substances emanating from the colon reach the hypothalamus by the blood stream when the colon has an accumulation of impacted noxious, toxic waste. To maintain your hypothalamus in a healthy, vigorous and energetic condition, watch what you eat, and particularly see to it that your eliminative system is clean.

It would take a whole volume to do justice to a comprehensive description of the ramifications of the Hypothalamus. I am emphasizing this in order to impress on you how very important it is to give the most meticulous care to every phase of your physical, mental and spiritual habits and attitudes in order that this vital center is your system may help you to attain and to maintain **VIBRANT HEALTH.**

Chapter 22
THE PITUITARY GLAND

The pituitary gland, divided into three specific lobes, is greatly controlled and regulated, as well as influenced, by the hypothalamus. It is classified in three sections, the anterior (or forward) pituitary, the posterior (or rearward) pituitary and the medial lobe of the pituitary.

The medial lobe of the pituitary is very small compared to the size of the rest of the gland. Its impact on the human race is terrific, inasmuch as it regulates and controls the male sperm in copulation in intercourse, influencing the type of the child-embryo. It usually reproduces the race of the male parent.

The anterior pituitary controls and regulates the secretion or generation of hormones in the thyroid, adrenal glands, liver, male and female organs, and in the secretion of insulin in the pancreas.

The posterior pituitary, also under the influence of the hypothalamus, regulates and controls the temperature of the body. This regulating mechanism is a miracle of complications, involving the blood temperature, the perspiration processes throughout the body, from head to foot, and the action of the pores of the skin which open during heat and close during cold environment.

The posterior pituitary also regulates the water balance in the body, an extremely important function when you realize that most of the body is composed of water. This function includes the constant exchange of water between, the blood and the tissues. The water in the system MUST therefore be kept clean and pure.

It is the function of the pituitary gland to regulate the excretion of water through the kidneys. In its temperature regulating operation the kidneys become more active in cold weather because the pores of the skin then close, preventing evaporation through the skin. In a hot environment, on the other hand, the pores open to release evaporation, hence there is a corresponding reduction in the activity of the kidneys.

The pituitary gland secretes or generates several distinct kinds of hormones. One hormone is concerned with the metabolism of proteins and carbohydrates, increasing glycogen production for heart and other muscles, and in the growth of bone and muscle.

Another hormone stimulates the secretion of the adrenal hormones.

Still another hormone stimulates the secretion and distribution of the thyroid hormones, and other hormones of equal activity and importance.

The most beneficial nourishment for the Pituitary Gland has been found to be the following vegetables, particularly when used in the form of juices, and either singly or in any of their combinations. Namely: Beets, carrots, cucumbers, celery and parsley. Fresh fruits in season are also good.

Chapter 23
THE ADRENAL GLANDS

The adrenal glands are two capsules resting on the top of the two kidneys. Their functions are as varied as they are vital.

The adrenal glands exert the regulatory functions of menstrual activity, and that of the reproductive glands. The regulation of the balance of certain atomic elements in the body, such as calcium, phosphorus chlorine and sodium, these last two particularly in their blood plasma content, come under the province of the adrenal glands. So do certain functions of the visual apparatus such as the dilation of the pupil of the eyes.

The adrenal glands are deeply involved in one's state of excitement and in one's emotions in connection with the solar plexus, a network of nerves right in the midriff.

As the adrenal glands regulate certain of the functions of peristalsis, their disfunction will cause intestinal disturbances, irritation and even greater discomforts. The disfunction of these glands is sometimes responsible for tumors, for low blood pressure and even for convulsions.

On the other hand, the adrenal glands have the effect of stimulating the muscles and the nerve systems as well as the repair and regeneration of cell and tissue structure.

Excessive coition, sexual copulation, has the effect of inhibiting and interfering with the activity of the hormone secretion and functions of the adrenal glands. This has a very disrupting effect on the entire system, from the brain, down.

The adrenal glands are a veritable mine, or fount of hormone secretions. They generate nearly four dozen different kinds and types of hormones. Nothing can be secreted or generated in the system without materials with which to constitute a substance. Consequently it is of vital importance, not only to furnish the body with food, but to supply it with nourishing food which can be assimilated quickly. There is no nourishment which is more perfectly adapted to the human system and particularly to its Endocrine Glands, than the fresh raw vegetable juices. The Adrenal Glands have been greatly benefited by drinking carrot juice and combinations of carrot - beet - and - coconut, carrot - lettuce - alfalfa and carrot and parsley juices. Special emphasis is placed on the green juices. These of course are made fresh from raw vegetables. Eating ripe papayas, when available, has also been most beneficial in maintaining the balanced activities of the adrenal glands.

Each of the two adrenal glands is enclosed in a little sack or capsule consisting of two definite and distinct layers. The inner layer is the Medulla, the outer layer is the Cortex.

The blood supply through the medulla is greater in daily volume than that through any other gland of a relative size in the body with the exception of the thyroid gland. The function of the medulla is the secretion of the hormones Epinephrine and Norepinephrine frequently labeled emergency hormones. They cause a rise in the blood pressure, a constriction of the blood vessels and acceleration of the heart.

The epinephrine hormone causes the release of sugar from the liver raising the blood sugar level.

The Cortex is of indispensable value to life. The cortex hormones make it possible for the body to meet conditions of intense emotional excitement and muscular exertion, of the stress of pain, shock and temperature extremes.

The preparation from the processing of glandular cortex in known as Cortisone, one of the most dangerous medications in attempting to cure disorders such as arthritis, if provision is not made to counteract its deleterious effects.

The pituitary gland secretes a hormone known as ACTH, short for adrenocorticotrophic hormone, which exerts a direct influence on the secretion of the hormones of the adrenal cortex. When Cortisone is used incorrectly or erroneously it can disrupt the smooth interaction between the pituitary and the adrenal glands, causing serious disturbances in the system.

Too much stress cannot be placed on the importance of caring for the body from every angle, physical, mental and spiritual. Neglect in any phase leads to ultimate disaster. The Endocrine Glands have been given to us for us to love, honor and obey them, so that our life may be lived more abundantly and so that we may attain and maintain **VIBRANT HEALTH.**

Chapter 24
THE THYROID GLAND

The thyroid gland is the largest of the Endocrine Glands, except the liver. It is the gland regulating the temperamental aspect in relation to the individual's disposition, nature, character, moods, peculiarities, and idiosyncrasies.

The thyroid is located in front and alongside Adam's apple in the throat. When you realize that every drop of blood in the body flows through the thyroid gland every quarter of an hour or so, and that every good and bad atomic and bacterial element is carried in the blood, you must appreciate why the thyroid has such a far reaching influence on young and old alike.

There are two atomic elements which are essential in the effective functioning of the thyroid, namely: iodine and zinc. If these elements, or either one, is deficient or lacking in the diet, the thyroid cannot obtain them from the blood as the blood flows through it. This results in a train of disturbances which interfere seriously with the individuals well-being and with his aim and desire to attain **VIBRANT HEALTH.**

The thyroid secretes or generates the hormone known as Thyroxine in the constitution of which both iodine and zinc are involved. Microscopic amounts of this thyroxine are picked up by the blood as it passes through the thyroid regulating many of its body functions, such as the metabolism of carbohydrates, the body's water balance, the functions of the various circulatory systems, the muscles, the nerves and the sex organs.

One of the paramount, essentially vital functions of the thyroid is in its reciprocal activities with the other Endocrine Glands, and the activities of the pituitary and adrenal glands in particular. A deficiency of zinc and iodine in the system results in the faulty metabolism of fats with the consequent building up of fatty adipose tissues where they are least wanted.

When this has been the case, the deficiency of iodine has been helped by the use of sea lettuce (leaf dulse), kelp and pure filtered ocean sea water.

The zinc deficiency has been helped by using zinc "tissue salts" in 6x potency, obtained from any Homeopathic Pharmacy, in tiny white round tablets, using four of these two or three times a day for a few weeks. These tablets are neither drugs nor medicine. They are mineral elements in the most easily assimilable form to help the mineral balance of the body.

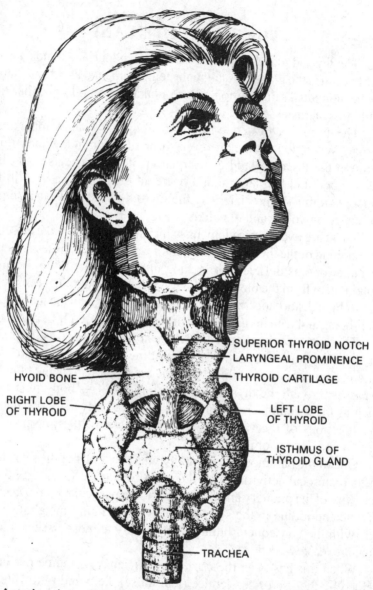

HYOID BONE

RIGHT LOBE
OF THYROID

SUPERIOR THYROID NOTCH
LARYNGEAL PROMINENCE

THYROID CARTILAGE

LEFT LOBE
OF THYROID

ISTHMUS OF
THYROID GLAND

TRACHEA

Anterior view of thyroid gland, showing its relationship to
the hyoid and trachea.

The overproduction by the thyroid of the thyroxine hormone
causes many kinds of disturbances such as goiters, loss of weight
resulting in emaciation, nervousness, restlessness, irritability, loss of
mental and physical vigor and the lowering of the rate of metabolism.

These conditions are equally helped by the judicious use of seaweeds and zinc, and fresh raw vegetable juices.

In any case, the best results have been obtained when a series of colon irrigations were used.

The value and the need of colon irrigations is a subject requiring meticulous attention, at least at periodic intervals. The toxins which corruption in the colon can generate are truly unbelievable if the individual has failed to study and consider this important matter. The glandular system of the body is the means by which all functions and activities of the body are made possible. Any disturbance or interference with their smooth operation cannot fail to have repercussions on the individual's well-being, and no phase of a person's daily life is more susceptible to the effects of toxemia than the glands.

Decomposition of waste, decayed feces tainted by pathogenic bacteria cannot by any stretch of the imagination induce a healthy environment. Right? The removal of corruption from the colon is just as vital, if not more so, than the removal of garbage from City Streets. Unless such corruption is removed from the colon, its putrefactive odors manifest as bad offensive breath and "body odors". Deodorants of any kind and nature whatever cannot hide, conceal or screen from the consciousness of people close by the fact that uncleanness, foulness and fetidness clog up the victim's system. The cleaner your own system is, the more obnoxious are odoriferous people around you.

This retention of corruption is of particularly vital importance in the case of the thyroid, because end-products of such corruption do seep into the blood and are thereby carried through the thyroid, leaving noxious deposits to generate afflicting disturbances.

The most important nourishing supplement to help maintain the balance of the thyroid is the iodine contained in seaweed. We use kelp or leaf dulse (sea lettuce) at nearly every meal.

Another invaluable adjunct, particularly to juices and other beverages, is pure filtered ocean Sea Water which contains all of the trace elements in the constitution of the human anatomy. Only a few drops of Sea Water are needed in any beverage.

Chapter 25
THE PINEAL GLAND

As explained in a preceding chapter, the Pineal Gland is undoubtedly the spiritual receptacle of the life force emanating from the Cosmic Energy of the Universe. Everything in the Universe exists because and by virtue of Cosmic Energy, the very essence of life. The tiny atom has its Cosmic Energy established in its constantly active electron.

The pineal is such a small gland that scientists failed to assign any importance to it until the last 40 years, and even today its mental and spiritual significance is not appreciated by the strict materialist.

The pineal hormone exerts a regulatory effect on both the pituitary gland and on the adrenal glands. When its secretion is excessive it results in the enlargement of these glands. When it is deficient it affects the pituitary hormone which can cause large areas of the skin to lose their natural color pigment.

The mental and spiritual influence of the pineal surpasses that of any other gland. It would almost seem as if this influence is directly connected with the relationship of the physical body of the individual and that mysterious and intangible part known as the soul.

By analogy this can perfectly well be the case. The "voltage" of Cosmic Energy surpasses any volume and strength which humans can obtain by any electrical or mechanical contrivances. If this terrifically powerful Cosmic Energy were to enter the body without control and reduction, the result would be like being struck by a bolt of lightning. As it is, the Thalamus gets the full impact of this Cosmic voltage and is the transformer which reduces the voltage to exactly the amount, volume and strength which the individual can withstand.

Basically, such attributes as stamina, energy, vigor and the like have their inception and are based upon the relative sensitiveness of the pineal-thalamus relationship.

It is very significant that the pineal gland is directly involved in the regulation of the reproductive organs in both male and female, as the propagation of the species, of the race, is the most important function of human beings.

Disfunction or incompetence of pineal hormone secretion results in the over-distension or decrease of the human height.

One of the most valuable foods for the nourishment of the pineal gland is the ripe papaya when taken with fresh raw carrot juice. This combination is one of the most normalizing for the entire human system.

Chapter 26
THE THYMUS GLAND

The importance of the Thymus Gland lies in its protective function against the invasion into the human system of excessive volumes of pathogenic, infectious organisms. The hormone secreted by the thymus gland stimulates the activity of the blood in the spleen activating the production of lymphocites to filter debris and bacteria. This stimulation extends to the lymph glands where lymphocites are constantly produced as scavenger organisms.

The thymus gland regulates the growth of the sex glands. It also regulates sexual activity.

So intimately is the thymus involved in the growth and development of the sex glands, that upon the reproductive organs reaching maturity after adolescence, the thymus gradually shrinks until little more than tissues remain. Nevertheless, its influence continues to function in its field of body activities.

Chapter 27
THE SEX GLANDS
(THE REPRODUCTIVE ORGANS)

The sex organs have been provided by Nature for the sole and specific purpose of reproducing the species.

Because of their extreme sensitivity, humanity, unlike the members of the animal kingdom, has used and abused the reproductive organs shamelessly.

The effect of the regulation, stimulation and disfunction of these glands has its impact on every phase of human existence, as these glands influence, regulate and control the functions and activities of nearly every gland in the body.

The mammary glands. The main function of these glands, which are located in the breast, is for the secretion of milk. Their activities, however, extend to assisting the regulation of the adrenal glands, the parathyroids, the thyroid and the sex glands. They regulate the assimilation of the carbon element in the food.

When healthy, they regulate menstruation, whereas when they fail to function normally, either scanty or excessive menstruation results. When the mammary glands are afflicted, the affliction affects all the reproductive organs.

The removal of breasts may result in the disturbance of the foregoing normal activities and functions. The patient sometimes realizes that surgery was a mistake. It is my considered opinion that breasts should never be removed, any more than any other gland that our Creator considered was needed in the human system.

When reproductive glands and organs are afflicted there arises the predisposition to the development of cysts or tumors, the mental balance and faculties suffer, dejection, melancholy, despondency, gloom and pessimism overcome the victim. The disfunction of the reproductive organs or glands also results in nervousness, irritability, impotency and excess adipose tissue.

To keep these glands functioning healthfully it is important to keep the body clean inside and out, and properly nourished with plenty of fresh raw vegetables and fruits and their juices.

A word of warning, here, is needed. Your thoughts have a direct influence on your body. You must have, or develop, wholesome thoughts, particularly when you are alone.

A clean, healthy mind and body are essential and indispensable elements for **VIBRANT HEALTH.**

Chapter 28

THE PROSTATE

THE PROSTATE GLAND regulates the seminal fluid and the generation of spermatozoa. It stimulates sex impulses when in a healthy condition, but when afflicted tends towards impotency.

About 40% of men who have reached the mid-century mark are more or less afflicted with prostate gland trouble. The prostate gland is the basic principle, the kernel, the essence of man's sexual life, and men base their masculine power, their strength and their virility on the efficiency of their sexual responses. Whatever happens to undermine and weaken his virile propensities causes anxiety, consternation and alarm.

The prostate gland is an organ with which every man should be thoroughly familiar regarding its purpose, its function, what causes it to be diseased and what he can and should do to prevent complications.

The prostate gland is a bulbular muscular organ the size of a walnut surrounding the neck of the bladder.

Through the center of the prostate gland there is a channel or duct about 3/16th of an inch diameter, known as the prostatic urethra, which is directly connected with the urinary bladder.

The prostate is a gland of internal and external secretion. It secretes a fluid which stimulates the activity of the sperm. The male germ, the spermatozoa, develops in the testes, is quiescent, motionless and is conveyed to the sperm-sack, known as the seminal vesicle, for storage, to await maturity. As and when the sperm is invested with the secretion of the prostate it becomes animated. The mixture of the secretion of the prostate with the sperm becomes the procreative semen.

The prostate is influenced by the middle lobe of the pituitary gland whereby the race-type and propensities of the male parent are usually reproduced, in the offspring, as the prototype of the father.

The secretion of the prostate also has the function of lubricating its central canal to protect it from any possible irritation when urine passes through it.

Another function of the prostate is to regulate the flow of urine from the bladder. The prostate keeps the outlet of the bladder tightly closed while the bladder is filling. When the need to urinate arrives, the prostate relaxes the outlet from the bladder and when the bladder is emptied the muscles of the prostate contract and expand to expel the urine which remains in the urinary canal.

Obviously any affliction of the prostate gland causes its first disturbance in the control of the urine in the bladder. This of course can lead to many complications and embarrassment.

The reproductive function of the prostate is to ensure pregnancy. If the channel through the prostate is inflamed man loses control of the ejaculation and the ejaculation is short-lived.

One of the primary causes of prostate trouble is the deliberate postponement of urination. This places a needless and excessive burden on the muscles of this gland which may result in inflammation and tendency to weaken its functions. Failure and neglect to empty the bladder when the consciousness has been awakened to this need will cause the pressure in the bladder to be considerably increased, resulting in congestion of the prostate.

Venereal disease has become such an epidemic throughout the world that all young and older people should be warned of the dreadful consequences of indulging in unprotected intercourse. Sexual promiscuity cannot lead to happiness nor to VIBRANT HEALTH, as you can never be confident of a complete cure from any sexually transmitted diseases.

As the rectum lies close to the prostate, every possibility of becoming constipated should be watched and avoided, as the excessive accumulation of feces in the rectum can readily cause so much pressure against the prostate that its functions and activities can be interfered with.

We have found that the daily habit of drinking one pint of the combination of carrot and spinach juice, and when possible a pint of carrot, beet and cucumber juice, much benefit has been derived to help both the constipation and the bladder troubles.

By maintaining these glands and organs functioning at their best, we can go a long way towards the attainment of **VIBRANT HEALTH.**

Let me inject a question here: Would it not be better to exercise self-discipline and mental and physical control in order to avoid these afflictions which can ruin the rest of your days and turn the rest of your life into a NIGHTMARE? Remember that THOUGHT PRECEDES THE ACT! Just keep this thought constantly in mind: **I WANT VIBRANT HEALTH!**

Chapter 29
VENEREAL DISEASES

While on the subject of venereal diseases, I am reminded of a terrific experience I had, as a very young man. I worked in an office. One day, the clerk whose desk was next to mine, came back from lunch looking as if he had literally been wrestling with a ghost. His face was as white as a sheet. He said to me: "Walker, I just had the most frightful education of my life. There is a wax-work exhibit at such and such a street - and if you have enough intestinal fortitude to be thoroughly shocked, and survive, I would suggest you go and see it."

This certainly aroused my curiosity, and as it was then my own lunch hour, I promptly followed his suggestion.

The exhibit was in a shop, the windows of which had been made opaque so that one could not look inside. I paid a shilling, and went in.

Along the walls and in the middle, parallel to the walls, were table after table. On each table was the full size reproduction of the various parts of the human anatomy, emphasizing particularly the reproductive organs of male and female. What shocked my system to its foundation were the wax models of diseased organs showing the ravages of gonorrhea and syphilis, the most disgusting, nauseating, offensive sight. Believe me, that was a lesson powerful enough to last me for the rest of my life.

A thousand times, since then, I have thought how perfectly wonderful and educational it would be if such an exhibit could be placed in every school in the country! I cannot imagine anything that would put the fear more into the heart and mind of boys and girls, as a wax exhibit such as that. Promiscuous sex activity would then certainly be on the wane.

Among the most revealing exhibits were those showing the interior of the organs. These were the ones showing the progress of the disease, in the male tracing the gradual erosion of the urinary tube passing through the prostate, eventually depriving it of its function to control the retention of urine. The ravages would creep into the urinary bladder and spread to the sheathing of the rectum in the course of a few years, disrupting both the urinary system and the regulation of the evacuation of excrement. In due course, the disease was shown to spread to the eyes, causing blindness, and when entering the bloodstream would result in affliction of serous membranes and of the synovial fluid in the joints, causing these to stiffen.

In the female organs exhibits it was strikingly demonstrated how difficult it is to diagnose the presence of the gonococcus until a long time after infection, because of the numerous analogous disturbances due to causes other than gonorrhea. Some of the diseases resulting from this infection are arthritis, affliction of the optic system sometimes resulting in total blindness, disfiguration of the skin, causing it to become horny and rough. Other complications indicated were severe swelling of the muscles, degeneration of the pleura (lungs), inflammation of the brain, disruption of the spinal cord, and hardening of the muscles of the heart.

Another table was covered with wax models of nearly all parts of the body which are afflicted with syphilis. This was truly devastating. It would be too sickening to go into all the details of the ravages wrought by this filthy disease. Perhaps the worst part of this disease is the difficulty of making an accurate diagnosis, because its clinical manifestations are legion and they can simulate those of almost any other disease.

Chapter 30
THE ANSWER
TO YOUR DILEMMA

Originally, man was created PERFECT. Our Creator created a perfect human in every respect.

Mankind was given freewill and was made a free moral agent. Our Creator never forces mankind to do anything. Our Creator made rules, statutes and commandments for the guidance of mankind.

Obviously mankind has chosen to violate these edicts, resulting in the present world chaos. The first world was made out of chaos; so, if we WANT to make a new world, we have the materials. Each one of us can do his share in changing the present state of lawlessness and disorder. It must begin with us, as individuals.

Every human being has a body equipped with the fighting ability to enable it to organize for mental and physical activity.

The jet-speed of today has come upon us almost over-night. Minutes fly into hours and days fly into months before man realizes the need to slow down, to relax, to survey his present in relation to the future he is aiming for. Man fails to shift into low gear frequently to meditate upon the road ahead on which he is traveling. The result is that the state of mental and physical action has become permanent. This causes man to be subjected to the vicissitudes of his environment, his surroundings and his daily labors.

This state of affairs contributes to the toll of failing health, worry, frustration and all the concomitant negative conditions and states of mind that lead to premature senility, decay, and an unduly early demise.

The human body still retains within it its inherent ability to readjust itself to a Natural living and nutritional regimen, if man will exert himself and make use of this ability to readjust his mental attitude towards his appetites and habits. The Laws of Nature are VERY SIMPLE. Eat mostly food in its raw state, preferably grown organically without chemical fertilizers and poison sprays. Breathe plentifully of all the fresh clean air you can find. Think POSITIVELY and thank your Creator for your waking up to these principles before you reach the point of no return.

It takes acres and acres to feed cattle and when one eats its flesh the eventual end-product is the accumulation of excessive amounts of uric acid in the system.

It only takes a comparatively small amount of land to grow all the vegetables and fruits that a family needs and the digestion of such food is constructive.

The most beneficial sweetening is honey. Two or three beehives on a few acres will enable the bees to collect their honey for miles around, and there is no sweetening product to compare to the value of honey as food.

Among the principles included in Natural Laws, thinking and emotions play a superlative part. A constantly joyful individual is not afflicted with negativity and frustrations. His mental clarity is enhanced. He is not readily overtaken with afflictions.

The solution to **VIBRANT HEALTH** is simple.

Chapter 31
ORGANICALLY GROWN FOOD.
ORGANIC GARDENING.

The word ORGANIC, when applied to vegetation, food, farming and agriculture, means that it is exhibiting characters peculiar to living organisms, pertaining to or derived from living organisms. Biologically, organisms are things or substances constituted to carry on the activities of life by means of live organs separate in function but mutually dependent. In other words, any living substance animal, vegetable, bacteria, etc., is an organism.

Obviously, nothing can be ORGANIC which does not exhibit or contain life. We cannot have life and death at one and the same time, but dead matter can certainly interfere with the expression and activities of life and of living substances.

There was a time, before this present mature generation was born, when most of the food available was more or less naturally organically grown. That is to say chemical fertilizers, which destroy the soil and its organic elements, were not yet generally available.

The basis of ORGANIC SOIL is the availability of the mineral and chemical live elements for plants in which their respective and corresponding enzymes are present in their most active and regenerative form.

Just as a builder of houses cannot construct them unless he has the material with which to build them, so with plants, they cannot be perfect, when the nutritional elements in vegetation are imperfect if they lack the contribution of organic matter needed for the growth and development of the roots.

Artificial chemical matter constituting chemical fertilizers has neither the power nor the ability to instill life in the soil. Their sole purpose is to speed up the growth of the plant and let the future take care of the consequences! Earthworms and soil bacteria shun these chemical substances, leaving the soil devoid of the very basic principle planned by Nature for the organic growth of vegetation. These chemicals "lock" the soil, hardening it.

Plants of every kind, grown in organically prepared soil are the most nutritious. If you are planting your garden or plan to do so, bear in mind that the more thoroughly composted soil has greater plant quality stimulant available, than a poorly composted one.

Humans, animals and plants nourished on food grown in well composted soil are able - all other things being equal - to resist disease. If for no other reason than this, every individual who can do so, should grow as much of his family's food in his own garden as possible, and so be able to control the quality of such nourishment.

It is not necessary to have a large piece of ground to grow organically all the food that a family can use throughout the year. It is very necessary that there should be a plentiful supply of water.

In order to have the soil efficiently capable to grow vegetation in an organically accepted manner, the two prerequisites are: (1) earthworms to fertilize the soil naturally with their castings, and aerate the soil. (2) The presence of an infinite number of live organisms in the form of soil bacteria to help break down the soil components and to disintegrate decayed and decomposed vegetation.

Under these conditions the plant roots can delve deeply into the soil to get the benefit of the Trace Elements which are usually deficient or missing in commercially fertilized soil.

The human body is composed of about 59 atomic mineral and chemical elements. In order to comply with the Law of Replenishment and Regeneration it is necessary that these elements be present in the food, and the food must obtain these elements organically from the soil.

16 of these elements are always in the constitution of vegetables, fruits, nuts and seeds, notwithstanding the fact that they may not be present 100% of their par standard. Nevertheless, the ability of the human body to overcome such a deficiency to a certain degree and within certain limitations, enables us to get by with the run-of-the-mill food available, such as it is.

The other 43 atomic elements, known as Trace Elements, however, are present in such infinitesimal microscopic amounts that usually many of them are deficient or missing in most of the vegetation grown on chemically fertilized soils. If for no other reason than to prevent such a deficiency, whoever is able to grow organically raised food should certainly do so, and in this way become sensitive to the value of the QUALITY of the food. Plants grown in organically composted soil can send their roots way down deep into the soil where they can find the Trace Elements. Chemical fertilizers "lock" up the soil, preventing the roots from delving where these Trace Elements are to be found.

All this is simple enough, because it is NATURAL.

The important question in these days revolves around the food which is available in our stores and supermarkets. Did you ever observe and study people selecting their purchase of vegetables and fruits from their shopping list, at the super-market displays of such produce? Watch them! So many people pick a handful of this and a handful of that, without reflection, observation and consideration, and stuff them into a bag and off they go. They have not the vaguest idea of the QUALITY of the food they are buying, and probably care less.

I have observed with interest that an amazing number of young people take their time to make their choice carefully, buying the freshest and best quality that is available.

It is fully time that housewives become informed about what constitutes QUALITY in food. After all, the intention, the purpose and the very idea of buying food is for the purpose of nourishing the body. Food cannot be completely nourishing if it is deficient in its essential constituents. Everybody desires HEALTH, VIBRANT HEALTH, and without knowing how to attain it they cannot allay the process of degeneration of the cells and tissues of the body which results in sickness and premature old age.

When housewives, en masse, demand organically grown high quality food it will be forthcoming. THAT will be the day when VIBRANT HEALTH will be within closer reach to a vast number of people who cannot imagine what is the matter with them now. In THAT DAY the markets will supply the QUALITY of the food we need.

Today we already see the salutary and beneficial outcome of the organic principles taught in the past few decades. Already many people, young and old, are getting back to the soil. Some are making the utmost use of the few square feet available in their yard. Some are even converting their lawns into vegetable gardens. Even people living in mobile homes use tiny plots of ground on which they grow many vegetables. Some are developing 50 feet by 150 feet plots of ground into flourishing food gardens. Others are going into larger gardening and farming projects with composting and organic planting methods which enable them to supply neighbors and stores with the surplus of the food beyond that required for their immediate families.

People who live in apartments need not be frustrated by lack of a garden. During World War II thousands of families all over the country formed gardening groups with friends and neighbors. They rented vacant unused land, they even used Park lands where available, and made flourishing vegetable and fruit gardens for their supply of fresh organically grown food.

Today we have a new kind of gardening which many people are enthusiastically engrossed in developing. It is known as "Kitchen Gardening". It consists of the sprouting of untreated seeds of many kinds and varieties. This method is very convenient for people who have no available soil to work with. This is a splendid means to obtain complete live nourishment to supplement the daily diet. This subject is covered in my book **DIET & SALAD SUGGESTIONS** under the caption "Sprouting Seeds".

Space, here, does not permit my elaborating this dissertation as fully as I would like to and as completely as it deserves. For purposes of education on this subject I would urge you to get and study J. I. Rodale's two books on the subject, namely;

HOW TO GROW VEGETABLES AND FRUITS BY THE ORGANIC METHOD,
and his
ENCYCLOPEDIA OF ORGANIC GARDENING.

Chapter 32
TRACE ELEMENTS AND
SEAWATER, DULSE AND KELP.

There is no soil on the face of the dry earth that is as rich and complete in essential mineral and chemical elements as the bottom of the oceans. For untold millions of years the top soil from mountain, valley and field has been washed by rain and snow directly and indirectly into the oceans.

Of all flesh food, fishes that have fins and scales, in rivers, lakes and the oceans, are among the most complete kind of edible flesh food which is suitable for man IF (note this IF) man chooses to eat flesh food. The reason for this is that fishes are born and have their being in the most nutritious healthy element on earth and that is SEA WATER. SEA WATER (that is, water from OCEANS but not from inland seas or lakes) contains all of the 59 atomic elements constituting the human body.

These elements consist of the 16 "gross" atomic elements present in the composition of vegetation, and the 43 Trace Elements usually elusive but of vital importance to the healthy maintenance of the human system. The following is the list of these 59 elements, (the 16 gross elements are indicated by *)

Actinium	Copper	Neptunium	*Silicon
Aluminum	Erbium	*Nitrogen	Silver
Argon	*Flourine	Osmium	*Sodium
Arsenic	Gold	*Oxygen	Strontium
Barium	*Hydrogen	*Phosphorus	*Sulfur
Bismuth	Indium	Platinum	Tantalum
Boron	*Iodine	Plutonium	Thallium
Bromine	Iridium	*Potassium	Thorium
*Calcium	*Iron	Radium	Thulium
*Carbon	Lanthanum	Rhenium	Tin
Caesium	Lead	Rubidium	Uranium
Cerium	Lithium	Ruthenium	Yttrium
*Chlorine	*Magnesium	Sarnarium	Zinc
Chromium	*Manganese	Scandium	Zinconium
Cobalt	Mercury	Selenium	

All these elements are present in the human body, provided that the individual in is perfect health .... But WHO IS in "perfect health"? The exigencies of present day civilized living make it virtually impossible for a person of any age, from a baby to a centenarian, to attain VIBRANT HEALTH by following the line of least resistance in the matter of food, drink, fresh air and exercise.

Something other than our present orthodox manner of living must be adopted and adopted with a considerable amount of urgency to stem the degeneration of the human body.

A healthy body is immune to disease by its very nature. Food is the means by which we keep body and spirit alive, and food is intended to furnish the body with all the live elements needed for the regeneration of its cells and tissues. If the body fails to be healthy, it is obvious that the lack or deficiency of regenerative elements in the food is the cause of, and the responsibility for, what ever ailment, sickness or disease overtakes it.

We have tried to prove to you in our preceding pages that no inorganic *solid* mineral or chemical substance can pass through or enter into the liver by the digestive processes, and be used for regeneration of the cells and tissues of the anatomy. Such minerals and chemicals can be furnished to the soil in their proper and natural state and the vegetation will convert them into colloidal or liquid substances which can nourish the body. All the mineral and chemical elements in SEA WATER are already in colloidal or liquid form and in their inherent state. In fact, they are so naturally concentrated that it requires only a minimal amount, actually a matter of a reasonably small number of drops, to vitalize and energize a whole tumblerful of fruit or vegetable juices. For example: oranges are not as good today as they were 20 or 30 years ago, because both soil and atmosphere have become too polluted for their good. We just bought a crate of oranges from a farmer who is both particular and fussy about his crops. We have bought oranges from him for years, but we have noticed, as the years went by, that there was a certain mild sting in their taste that became more pronounced of late, although the quality otherwise is excellent. By adding about a quarter teaspoonful or less of CATALINA SEA WATER to each tumblerful of orange juice the taste and quality was immediately enhanced, and we enjoyed a delicious drink.

As a matter of fact, we always keep a pint bottle of CATALINA SEA WATER (which we buy at the Health Food Store) in our kitchen and add a few drops from it to every beverage, even to pure straight water when we drink it, and to our salads and other food. In this way we feel confident that we are getting our quota of Trace Elements into our system every day.

You cannot conceive the very small microscopic amount of each trace element which the body must have in order to be VIBRANTLY HEALTHY. Some parts and functions of the body need only one or two Trace Elements. For example: The sinovial fluid, the lubricating substance in the joints, requires Bismuth. The outer skin of the body needs Chromium. The appendix needs Erbium. The pineal gland needs both Iridium and Lithium. Bone marrow requires Iron and Phosphorus. The kidneys need Iron and Neptunium. The gall bladder requires Neptunium.

The cerebro-spinal fluid needs Actinium, Bromine, Lanthanum, Oxygen, Radium and Uranium. The blood circulation of the brain requires Bromine, Oxygen, Platinum, Selenium and Thallium.

The list of parts and functions of the anatomy requiring their atomic Trace Elements in order to perform at maximum efficiency, and the various elements involved, is too long to include completely in this brief dissertation. The few examples I have cited should prove how important it is to keep the body constantly replenished with a supply of these invaluable, elusive Trace Elements, to attain **VIBRANT HEALTH.**

Sea vegetation, in the form of Dulse (sea lettuce), and kelp, in addition to the daily use of SEA WATER, should help to keep the system in sufficient balance to maintain a state of **VIBRANT HEALTH,** other things being equal. The elimination of waste matter from the body should be meticulously taken care of by means of enemas and colon irrigations whenever there is the slightest indication that the eliminative organs are becoming sluggish.

In this eliminative washing out process, do not be misled into the thought that they are not beneficial. Also disregard any claims that they cause the loss of intestinal flora, as this is not true. No intestinal flora can exist nor flourish when the fecal matter clogs up the glands in the colon that cause the flora to flourish. When the colon has been cleaned or washed out, then drinking a pint of the combination of carrot and spinach juice has been used successfully to help the intestinal flora to be fully re-established.

Of all the 59 Trace Elements we have found that ZINC is involved in nearly every function and activity of the human anatomy. There are Homeopathic Pharmacies in most of the large cities and you can no doubt obtain their name and address from the Yellow Pages of the Telephone Directories of the cities nearest to you. We obtain our supply of ZINC 6X in bottles containing 2,000 tablets, from the Standard Homeopathic Company in Los Angeles, California. We use the 6X potency and take four tablets at a time, usually dissolved in about ¼ cup of warm water or in a glass of vegetable juice. Or we may take them dry - once or twice a day - dissolving them on the tongue, followed by some vegetable juice. We feel that this keeps our Zinc balance up to par. We cannot depend on the Zinc content of the vegetables and fruits we buy.

Chapter 33
HEALTH AND HYGIENE.

During a Parliamentary debate in the British House of Commons in London around 1875, on the question of Public Health, Britain's Prime Minister, Benjamin Disraeli, declared:

"Public Health is the foundation on which repose the happiness of the people and the power of a country. The care of public health is the first duty of a statesman".

With all the knowledge which is available today about hygiene and cleanliness, one would expect scientists to attack the problem of sickness and disease at its source, that is, within the human organism, instead of outside of it.

Granted that maintaining communities in cleaner, more sanitary environment has helped to lower the death rate of communicable diseases, this step still leaves the individual susceptible to contagious afflictions in his environment if his intestinal tract is a magnet for parasites.

Whatever angle of the problem is attacked, it is today common knowledge that there is no more prolific feeding ground for pathogenic germs and bacteria than human excrement maintained at temperatures of 98° to 100° F (37° to 38° C) - body temperatures. This being the case, I have steadfastly maintained that the contents of the human colon is the first place to search for the CAUSE of any ailment, sickness or disease, and to proceed to clean out the colon instead of cutting any of it out.

Sickness does not spring upon a person "out of the blue". It is the cumulative effect of neglecting the fundamental principles of health and hygiene, and to maintain the eliminative organs thoroughly clean and properly nourished.

The fact has been generally overlooked that bugs, germs, and the like, need food to be able to exist. They are scavengers. Waste and corruption in the human body is the media on which they feed and propagate. Deprive them of food, and they die.

When the human body is kept clean of waste, debris and corruption there is nothing for them on which to feed. Consequently they die before propagating and causing trouble.

As an example, consider HEART TROUBLE! The failure to PREVENT more than three quarters of a million deaths from heart "trouble" each year is appalling. The human heart is the most miraculous, persistent, indefatigable contrivance ever devised, stronger than almost any other part of the human anatomy. It has to be, in order to pump more than 45 MILLION GALLONS of blood through the system in the span of a mere 50 years, with a DAILY heart-beat of some 100,000 "beats" a day. Methusaleh, the Patriarch of old, born in 3317 B.C., who died in 2348 B.C., the son of Enoch and the grandfather of Noah, had a heart that must have pumped 855 MILLION GALLONS of blood through his system, during his 960 years lifetime.

It is inconceivable that humanity's anatomy has degenerated to the point where three quarters of a million people died prematurely of heart "trouble" in just one year. Like a number of other Doctors, who disagree with the theory that the heart degenerates so early in life, I have found that the trouble with the heart usually stems from the corruption in the colon.

Many years ago I was in business with a gentleman only a year or two older than I. He was a gourmet and an epicure, no food was too good (or sufficient) for him. He ridiculed my way of eating and living, and we often had some strong discussions and arguments on the subject. His midriff advertised his way of living - by the bulge. The very mention of cleansing the colon would spark his irascibility and his temper would flare up. More than 40 years ago his death certificate read "Coronary Occlusion". The true and correct verdict would have been "Intestinal Occlusion and Putrefaction". Anyway, he died much too young, while I, today, 40 years later, am ALIVE, awake, alert and full of enthusiasm, thankful for my knowledge about the care of my body.

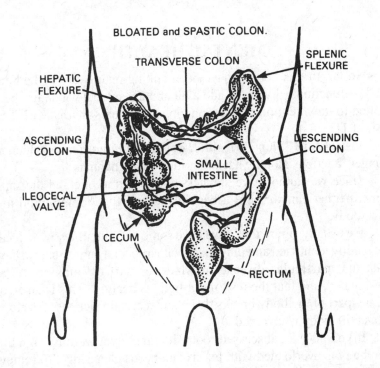

BLOATED and SPASTIC COLON.

TRANSVERSE COLON

SPLENIC FLEXURE

HEPATIC FLEXURE

ASCENDING COLON

DESCENDING COLON

SMALL INTESTINE

ILEOCECAL VALVE

CECUM

RECTUM

Just look at, and study, the accompanying illustration of a distorted colon. This is comparatively mild alongside many others, such as those in the vignettes on my Colon Therapy Chart in a preceding chapter.

VIBRANT HEALTH is the result of a system maintained meticulously clean, within and without the body properly nourished, and the Hypothalamus balanced, indicating the temperature, the temper and the temperament are all balanced and under perfect control.

Chapter 34
MENTAL HEALTH

So far, in this book, I have been talking mainly about the body and its functions. I want to add a bit about a subject which has been called to the attention of everyone in recent years-that is MENTAL HEALTH.

Just what IS "Mental Health"? It is a sick mind, a mind which no longer functions along what we term normal channels.

Since we cannot have sickness and health at one and the same time, neither can we have a healthy, normal functioning mind in a sick body.

We usually figure that if we have some definite illness which can be readily identified and diagnosed with a special name, that we have just that particular disease in whatever part of our body is so designated, and that the rest of our body is healthy. This is an error. If any part of the body breaks down and a certain sickness develops, the entire body is involved.

If you have an abscessed tooth, it is merely a warning sign that the body is overloaded with toxins and needs cleansing. To remove the tooth is dealing only with the effect, and not with the cause of the trouble. Cleansing and properly nourishing the body, eliminating from the diet, foods which have created the condition, and drinking an abundance of fresh raw vegetable juices daily, is a slower method of helping to relieve ourselves of the pain which we feel we cannot bear. It is the only sensible approach which we have discovered, to solve the problem satisfactorily.

There is a reaction for every action, and sometimes the reaction is delayed for such a long time that when it sets in, we do not connect it with the action which started it.

Since you cannot feed the body on garbage and expect to have **VIBRANT HEALTH,** neither can you feed the mind on garbage and expect to have a HEALTHY VIBRANT MIND!

All health begins in the home. If healthy parents beget healthy children and properly guide, direct, instruct and discipline them from infancy up, giving them loving care and good wholesome live food to build healthy disease-free bodies, they will grow up with healthy minds.

Our minds feed on what we hear and see around us, on what we are taught and on what we read. Until a child is old enough to start going to school, the parents are responsible for the available food that the young and tender mind feeds on. If a child is permitted to just grow up like a weed, with no special training in the home regarding - morals, manners, self-discipline and respect for the rights of others, that child starts out in life mentally crippled and handicapped, and has a slim chance of ever enjoying VIBRANT MENTAL HEALTH.

Regardless of age, all people have the tendency to want to imitate what others are doing, and this trait is particularly predominant in children. They will imitate what they see their parents do and say, whether good or bad.

If just one generation of parents could raise just one generation of children VIBRANTLY HEALTHY in body and mind, free from all sickness and disease, and train them to live clean, healthy, wholesome lives, how quickly could this sick world be transformed into a veritable literal GARDEN OF EDEN!

We all need to set a watchman at the door of our mind with a strict set of rules and regulations regarding what is allowed to pass into our mind, for once it is there we tend to think on it, and each one of us is a creator in that we are constantly creating our future life by what we see, hear, read, feel and think about. Our Creator gave you free will. It is entirely up to you to determine what you make of your life. Does it not seem that, knowing this, you should make every effort to choose the right way, so that you can be assured of VIBRANT HEALTH and a good life?

VIBRANT HEALTH cannot be counterfeited. Either YOU HAVE IT, or you do NOT have it!

Chapter 35
WHAT YOU SOW,
THAT WILL YOU REAP

A visitor was going through a prison, one day. He passed by a prisoner sitting on a bench using a needle sewing a patch on his prison uniform. By way of conversation the visitor asked the prisoner: "Are you sewing ?"

"No, replied the prisoner, I'm REAPING!"

How true that is in everything in life. What we sow, that is what we will reap. Every good has its reward, every evil its penalty.

This is probably one of the hardest and most difficult lessons we have had to learn from earliest childhood.

This important fact must be instilled in the consciousness of every growing child, in the home. This principle must be instilled into the minds of children daily by their parents in order that the fact and its impression will be indelibly sculptured into the consciousness of the growing child.

Just as the drip-drip-dripping of water will wear away a stone, so also the constant daily repetition of this lesson from parent to child will tend to avoid the many physical and mental afflictions which beset us later in life.

In the matter of **VIBRANT HEALTH** it is far better to attain it by disciplining the appetites than to wish for it and envy those who have it. Personal effort is involved.

VIBRANT HEALTH is the outcome of constant attention to discipline. Discipline of the mind and thoughts. Discipline of the emotions. Discipline of the kind and type of pleasure and indulgences. Discipline of the appetites and the desires of the flesh.

The selection of food is a discipline which requires careful thought, attention and choice. The human body thrives on the simplicity of its nourishment. The life principle in what we eat begets life development in the cells and tissues of the body. Such life is the foundation for **VIBRANT HEALTH.**

The truly **VIBRANTLY HEALTHY** body does not desire drugs, false stimulants, nor anything else that will disrupt the even tenor of its functions and activities.

When you sow the right kind of nourishment into your body, and at the same time meticulously watch the elimination of waste, you reap **VIBRANT HEALTH.**

When you have learned to banish from your consciousness all and every resentment that developed within you since you were born, when you have learned to be in complete control of your emotions, then, in addition to **VIBRANT HEALTH,** you will have learned to be in control of life, instead of letting life control you.

When you are young and inexperienced you never want to hear or take advice from those older than yourself. You feel that you want to experience everything personally.

To be young and full of enthusiasm is in itself a great experience, but it is not the experience that is required in the management of life and its affairs.

It is a great mistake to think that experience can be obtained by wishful thinking. Experience means actually living through events, personally undergoing something in general as it occurs. It means anything that has been lived through.

Experience embodies all that has happened to one, everything that one has seen or done. Experience is the effect of something that has happened to one, the individual's reaction to events and to feelings.

Experience embodies the activities that include training, observation of practice and personal participation, knowledge, skill and the practice resulting from these.

Wishful thinking does not beget experience.

What better conclusion on the subject of experience can you arrive at, than AS YOU SOW, SO SHALL YOU REAP.

Chapter 36
DR. WALKER'S PROGRAM
TO A HEALTHIER MORE VIBRANT LIFE

Raw vegetable and fruit juices offer all the live enzymes and detoxicating qualities needed to keep our bodies strong, healthy and able to combat the many enemies of contamination and pollution in the world today. Our immune systems are kept at their peak when we consume "raw" vegetable and fruit juices on a daily basis. Vegetable juices are the "builders" of the body, while fruit juices are the "cleansers". Every cell, gland and organ benefits from pure, natural form of nutrition. It is comforting to realize that by drinking raw vegetable and fruit juices every day, our diet is complete in all the vitamins and minerals it needs to remain younger, stronger and healthier.

"Fresh Vegetable and Fruit Juices" by Dr. N. W. Walker was written to better explain the emphasize the procedures and specific benefits of juicing. Raw carrot juice for instance is rich in Vitamins A, B, B, C, D, E, and K. Properly prepared raw carrot juice aids digestion and is valuable in the maintenance of the bone structure that supports our entire body, including the teeth. Even intestinal and liver diseases are sometimes due to the lack of certain vitamins and minerals found in raw carrot juice. Endive juice contains elements essential to the optic systems while the cucumber juice offers the best of diuretic qualities. The list goes on.

It is well worth ones time to study the benefits derived from "fresh raw" juices. Actually, it's worth far more than your time . . . after all, this is your health and your life. Take control, feel better, look younger, and enjoy your life more completely. You are worth it!

Keep the colon clean. The health of your colon can be an indicator of your health. Laxatives are not healthy and certainly not the proper answer to constipation. Raw vegetable salads, fresh fruits, legumes and unprocessed grains along with plenty of distilled water will keep your colon regular and healthy. "Colonic Irrigations" once or twice a year, along with enemas done at home, offer an optimum way in which to insure a clean and active, healthy intestinal track. Being "regular" is having a bowel movement at least once a day, though often times two or three movements a day is ideal. The elimination of red meat and all processed foods from the diet is equally important. A well cleansed colon in perfect working order is absolutely essential for a long, productive and active life. It is important to note that when the colon is healthy, and not blocked, you are avoiding innumerable ailments. Because the colon is a natural breeding ground for pathogenic bacteria, it is essential that we prevent a toxic condition from developing in the colon. By maintaining a proper and clean environment for the "good bacteria" we avoid the "bad bacteria" which is dangerous and disease producing.

Drink PURE water. The body is dependent on fresh, clean water. The minerals, bacteria, and commercial additives in inorganic water (i.e. tap, spring, well water, etc.) are inorganic and cannot be utilized by the body. The vitamins and minerals within vegetables and fruits and their juices are organic and therefore beneficial to your health. Distilled water is in reality steam that has condensed back into water. Bacteria, parasites (including Cryptosporidium parvum that is so devastating to those in ill health) is destroyed by the distillation process. Some authorities believe that distilled water acts like a "sponge" and assits the body in eliminating toxins, etc. through the body's normal elimination processes. Drink plenty of vegetable and fruit juices and pure water.

Regular exercise. It keeps our hearts healthy, our blood pressure intact, our respiratory systems strong, and our metabolism balanced. Walking is the best exercise you can do. It can burn calories and tone muscles. In addition to weight control, exercise strengthens the immune system, relieves stress, and because of the release of endorphins, lifts your spirits. Recent medical research as found that during exercise the body releases several different chemicals, some of which have been found to deter cancer. A 30-minute walk every day is truly beneficial to your health. Also, bear in mind that the body needs sufficient rest and sleep to function at its' best.

Control your weight. Weight control is a very real and all to common problem among Americans today. Carrying an excess amount of weight dramatically affects the state of ones overall health. High blood pressure, clogged arteries and fatigue are only a few reasons why maintaining a healthy weight is so imperative. A long and healthy life cannot be achieved when the body is forced to deal with such a myriad of dilemmas. Weight control need not even be an issue if we simply restrict our food consumption to salads composed of raw vegetables and fruits, drink their juices and distilled water. You will feel much healthier and your vitality will increase, when all red meats, fats, commercial sugars and starches are eliminated from the diet.

The elimination of unhealthy products. Some of the most harmful food products consumed today include processed sugars, harmful fats, cow's milk and soft drinks. Because the human body does not tolerate, and in many cases, is damaged from the consumption of such products, one would be wise to consider not ingesting them. This elimination may very well in and of itself, better insure a longer and healthier life. The pancreas, for instance, is both overworked and subject to disturbing reactions when we consume sugar. When the body processes meat it produces a great deal of uric acid. The muscles absorb much of what should be expelled through the eliminative system and what sometimes occurs is the manifestation of various conditions such as rheumatism, neuritis and sciatic. It is self-preserving not to tempt bad health with bad food choices.

Alcohol and tobacco products are carcinogenic, organ damaging and life threatening to all who imbibe. Though these habits remain widespread throughout our world today, few would argue of their obvious dangers to our health and to the negative effect on the very length of life itself. To live longer, healthier and with vitality, we should eliminate all detrimental products from our lives.

Other vital nutrients that play important defense roles in your health include plentiful amounts of Vitamin C, raw onions and garlic. They offer strong immune boosting qualities, act as an excellent cleansing agents, are readily available, and should be taken advantage of on a regular basis. Ideally we would all grow our own food in our own healthy soil. But this of course, is not an option for the majority of our population. What is possible is selecting the best of all foods that you can possibly find.

Last, but not least, is our spiritual and emotional health. Stress, anger, resentment, the need to "get even" are all negative emotions and can play havoc with our physical health. Heart attacks, strokes and nervous disorders are only a few of the conditions associated with such a negative lifestyle. The opposite of negativism is optimism. Laughter, spiritual strength, the ability to forgive and forget, to deal with our every day problems with an attitude of solving them is essential to keep the glands in our body working together. Our physical health is dependent upon a calm, serene mental attitude.

In Conclusion. Self-preservation utilizes wisdom. The knowledge and application of defensive procedures can do much to protect and lengthen our lives. For instance, it is as wise to always wear a seatbelt as it is to avoid preservatives and pollutants whenever possible. Adopting and exchanging unhealthy habits to healthy habits is as easy as eating smaller meals, eating them more frequently, and chewing ones' food for a longer period of time are changes your entire digestive system will thank you for. Utilize your wisdom, it will benefit you greatly in your quest to live a long and vibrant life.

APPENDIX:

For one who is not accustomed to the use of Fahrenheit or Centigrade Thermometers, it is always confusing to figure out, for example, what the Centigrade temperature reading is, compared to the familiar Fahrenheit Temperature reading. For this reason I have inserted here these respective Conversion Tables showing:

Inches into Centimeters,
Centimeters into Inches,
Feet into Meters,
Meters into Feet,
Cubic Feet into Liters,
Liters into Cubic Feet,

U.S. Gallons into Liters,
Liters into U.S. Gallons,
Centigrade into Fahrenheit,
Fahrenheit into Centigrade,
Millimeters into Inches,

WEIGHTS AND MEASURES

Inches into Centimeters

Inches	0 Cm.	1 Cm.	2 Cm.	3 Cm.	4 Cm.	5 Cm.	6 Cm.	7 Cm.	8 Cm.	9 Cm.
0	......	2.54	5.08	7.62	10.16	12.70	15.24	17.78	20.32	22.86
10	25.40	27.94	30.48	33.02	35.56	38.10	40.64	43.18	45.72	48.26
20	50.80	53.34	55.88	58.42	60.96	63.50	66.04	68.58	71.12	73.66
30	76.20	78.74	81.28	83.82	86.36	88.90	91.44	93.98	96.52	99.06
40	101.60	104.14	106.68	109.22	111.76	114.30	116.84	119.38	121.92	124.46
50	127.00	129.54	132.08	134.62	137.16	139.70	142.24	144.78	147.32	149.86
60	152.40	154.94	157.48	160.02	162.56	165.10	167.64	170.18	172.72	175.26
70	177.80	180.34	182.88	185.42	187.96	190.50	193.04	195.58	198.12	200.66
80	203.20	205.74	208.28	210.82	213.36	215.90	218.44	220.98	223.52	226.06
90	228.60	231.14	233.68	236.22	238.76	241.30	243.84	246.38	248.92	251.46
100	254.00	256.54	259.08	261.62	264.16	266.70	269.24	271.78	274.32	276.86

Centimeters into Inches

Cm.	0 Inch	1 Inch	2 Inch	3 Inch	4 Inch	5 Inch	6 Inch	7 Inch	8 Inch	9 Inch
0	......	0.394	0.787	1.181	1.575	1.969	2.362	2.756	3.150	3.543
10	3.937	4.331	4.724	5.118	5.512	5.906	6.299	6.693	7.087	7.480
20	7.874	8.268	8.662	9.055	9.449	9.843	10.236	10.630	11.024	11.418
30	11.811	12.205	12.599	12.992	13.386	13.780	14.173	14.567	14.961	15.355
40	15.748	16.142	16.536	16.929	17.323	17.717	18.111	18.504	18.898	19.292
50	19.685	20.079	20.473	20.867	21.260	21.654	22.048	22.441	22.835	23.229
60	23.622	24.016	24.410	24.804	25.197	25.591	25.985	26.378	26.772	27.166
70	27.560	27.953	28.347	28.741	29.134	29.528	29.922	30.316	30.709	31.103
80	31.497	31.890	32.284	32.678	33.071	33.465	33.859	34.253	34.646	35.040
90	35.434	35.827	36.221	36.615	37.009	37.402	37.796	38.190	38.583	38.977
100	39.370	39.764	40.158	40.552	40.945	41.339	41.733	42.126	42.520	42.914

Feet into Meters

Feet	0 Meters	1 Meters	2 Meters	3 Meters	4 Meters	5 Meters	6 Meters	7 Meters	8 Meters	9 Meters
0	......	0.305	0.610	0.914	1.219	1.524	1.829	2.134	2.438	2.743
10	3.048	3.353	3.658	3.962	4.267	4.572	4.877	5.182	5.486	5.791
20	6.096	6.401	6.706	7.010	7.315	7.620	7.925	8.229	8.534	8.839
30	9.144	9.449	9.753	10.058	10.363	10.668	10.972	11.277	11.582	11.887
40	12.192	12.496	12.801	13.106	13.411	13.716	14.020	14.325	14.630	14.935
50	15.239	15.544	15.849	16.154	16.459	16.763	17.068	17.373	17.678	17.983
60	18.287	18.592	18.897	19.202	19.507	19.811	20.116	20.421	20.726	21.031
70	21.335	21.640	21.945	22.250	22.555	22.859	23.164	23.469	23.774	24.079
80	24.383	24.688	24.993	25.298	25.602	25.907	26.212	26.517	26.822	27.126
90	27.431	27.736	28.041	28.346	28.651	28.955	29.260	29.565	29.870	30.174
100	30.479	30.784	31.089	31.394	31.698	32.003	32.308	32.613	32.918	33.222

Meters into Feet

Meters	0 Feet	1 Feet	2 Feet	3 Feet	4 Feet	5 Feet	6 Feet	7 Feet	8 Feet	9 Feet
0	.....	3.281	6.562	9.842	13.123	16.404	19.685	22.966	26.247	29.527
10	32.808	36.089	39.370	42.651	45.932	49.212	52.493	55.774	59.055	62.336
20	65.617	68.897	72.178	75.459	78.740	82.021	85.302	88.582	91.863	95.144
30	98.425	101.71	104.99	108.27	111.55	114.83	118.11	121.39	124.67	127.95
40	131.23	134.51	137.79	141.08	144.36	147.64	150.92	154.20	157.48	160.76
50	164.04	167.32	170.60	173.88	177.16	180.45	183.73	187.01	190.29	193.57
60	196.85	200.13	203.41	206.69	209.97	213.25	216.53	219.82	223.10	226.38
70	229.66	232.94	236.22	239.50	242.78	246.06	249.34	252.62	255.90	259.19
80	262.47	265.75	269.03	272.31	275.59	278.87	282.15	285.43	288.71	291.99
90	295.27	298.56	301.84	305.12	308.40	311.68	314.96	318.24	321.52	324.80
100	328.08	331.36	334.64	337.93	341.21	344.49	347.77	351.05	354.33	357.61

Cubic Feet into Liters (Cubic Decimeters)

Cubic Feet	0 Liters	1 Liters	2 Liters	3 Liters	4 Liters	5 Liters	6 Liters	7 Liters	8 Liters	9 Liters
0	.....	28.32	56.63	84.95	113.26	141.58	169.89	198.21	226.53	254.84
10	283.16	311.47	339.79	368.11	396.42	424.74	453.06	481.37	509.69	538.00
20	566.32	594.64	622.95	651.27	679.58	707.90	736.22	764.53	792.85	821.16
30	849.48	877.80	906.11	934.43	962.74	991.06	1019.4	1047.7	1076.0	1104.3
40	1132.6	1160.8	1189.2	1217.5	1245.9	1274.2	1302.5	1330.8	1359.1	1387.4
50	1415.8	1444.0	1472.4	1500.7	1529.1	1557.4	1585.7	1614.0	1642.3	1670.6
60	1698.9	1727.2	1755.5	1783.8	1812.2	1840.5	1868.8	1897.1	1925.4	1953.7
70	1982.1	2010.3	2038.7	2067.0	2095.4	2123.7	2152.0	2180.3	2208.6	2236.9
80	2265.3	2293.5	2321.9	2350.2	2378.6	2406.9	2435.2	2463.5	2491.8	2520.1
90	2548.4	2576.6	2605.0	2633.3	2661.6	2690.0	2718.3	2746.6	2774.9	2803.2
100	2831.6	2859.8	2888.2	2916.5	2944.9	2973.2	3001.5	3029.8	3058.1	3086.4

Liters (Cubic Decimeters) into Cubic Feet

Liters	0 Cubic Feet	1 Cubic Feet	2 Cubic Feet	3 Cubic Feet	4 Cubic Feet	5 Cubic Feet	6 Cubic Feet	7 Cubic Feet	8 Cubic Feet	9 Cubic Feet
0	.....	0.0353	0.0706	0.1059	0.1413	0.1766	0.2119	0.2472	0.2825	0.3178
10	0.3531	0.3884	0.4237	0.4590	0.4944	0.5297	0.5540	0.6003	0.6356	0.6709
20	0.7063	0.7416	0.7766	0.8122	0.8476	0.8829	0.9182	0.9535	0.9888	1.0241
30	1.0594	1.0947	1.1300	1.1653	1.2007	1.2360	1.2713	1.3066	1.3419	1.3772
40	1.4126	1.4479	1.4832	1.5185	1.5539	1.5892	1.6245	1.6608	1.6951	1.7304
50	1.7658	1.8011	1.8364	1.8717	1.9071	1.9424	1.9777	2.0130	2.0483	2.0836
60	2.1189	2.1542	2.1895	2.2248	2.2602	2.2955	2.3308	2.3661	2.4014	2.4367
70	2.4721	2.5074	2.5427	2.5780	2.6134	2.6487	2.6840	2.7193	2.7546	2.7899
80	2.8252	2.8605	2.8958	2.9311	2.9665	3.0018	3.0371	3.0724	3.1077	3.1430
90	3.1784	3.2137	3.2490	3.2843	3.3197	3.3550	3.3903	3.4256	3.4609	3.4962
100	3.5315	3.5668	3.6021	3.6374	3.6728	3.7081	3.7434	3.7787	3.8140	3.8493

U. S. Gallons into Liters

Gallons	0 Liters	1 Liters	2 Liters	3 Liters	4 Liters	5 Liters	6 Liters	7 Liters	8 Liters	9 Liters
0	.....	3.785	7.571	11.356	15.142	18.927	22.713	26.498	30.283	34.069
10	37.854	41.640	45.425	49.211	52.996	56.781	60.567	64.352	68.138	71.923
20	75.709	79.494	83.280	87.065	90.850	94.636	98.421	102.21	105.99	109.78
30	113.56	117.35	121.13	124.92	128.70	132.49	136.28	140.06	143.85	147.63
40	151.42	155.20	158.99	162.77	166.56	170.34	174.13	177.92	181.70	185.49
50	189.27	193.06	196.84	200.63	204.41	208.20	211.98	215.77	219.56	223.34
60	227.13	230.91	234.70	238.48	242.27	246.05	249.84	253.62	257.41	261.19
70	264.98	268.77	272.55	276.34	280.12	283.91	287.69	291.48	295.26	299.05
80	302.83	306.62	310.41	314.19	317.98	321.76	325.55	329.33	333.12	336.90
90	340.69	344.47	348.26	352.05	355.83	359.62	363.40	367.19	370.97	374.76
100	378.54	382.33	386.11	389.90	393.69	397.47	401.26	405.04	408.83	412.61

Liters into U. S. Gallons

Liters	0 Gallons	1 Gallons	2 Gallons	3 Gallons	4 Gallons	5 Gallons	6 Gallons	7 Gallons	8 Gallons	9 Gallons
0	.....	0.264	0.528	0.793	1.057	1.321	1.585	1.849	2.113	2.378
10	2.642	2.906	3.170	3.434	3.698	3.963	4.227	4.491	4.755	5.019
20	5.283	5.548	5.812	6.076	6.340	6.604	6.868	7.133	7.397	7.661
30	7.925	8.189	8.453	8.718	8.982	9.246	9.510	9.774	10.038	10.303
40	10.567	10.831	11.095	11.359	11.623	11.888	12.152	12.416	12.680	12.944
50	13.209	13.473	13.737	14.001	14.265	14.529	14.794	15.058	15.322	15.586
60	15.850	16.114	16.379	16.643	16.907	17.171	17.435	17.699	17.964	18.228
70	18.492	18.756	19.020	19.284	19.549	19.813	20.077	20.341	20.605	20.869
80	21.134	21.398	21.662	21.926	22.190	22.454	22.719	22.983	23.247	23.511
90	23.775	24.040	24.304	24.568	24.832	25.096	25.360	25.625	25.889	26.153
100	26.417	26.681	26.945	27.210	27.474	27.738	28.002	28.266	28.530	28.795

Comparison Between Degrees Centigrade and Degrees Fahrenheit

Deg. C.	Deg. F.	Deg. C.	Deg. F.	Deg. C.	Deg. F.	Deg. C.	Deg. F.	Deg. C.	Deg. F.	Deg. C.	Deg. F.
-40	-40.0	8	46.4	56	132.8	104	219.2	152	305.6	200	392.0
-39	-38.2	9	48.2	57	134.6	105	221.0	153	307.4	201	393.8
-38	-36.4	10	50.0	58	136.4	106	222.8	154	309.2	202	395.6
-37	-34.6	11	51.8	59	138.2	107	224.6	155	311.0	203	397.4
-36	-32.8	12	53.6	60	140.0	108	226.4	156	312.8	204	399.2
-35	-31.0	13	55.4	61	141.8	109	228.2	157	314.6	205	401.0
-34	-29.2	14	57.2	62	143.6	110	230.0	158	316.4	206	402.8
-33	-27.4	15	59.0	63	145.4	111	231.8	159	318.2	207	404.6
-32	-25.6	16	60.8	64	147.2	112	233.6	160	320.0	208	406.4
-31	-23.8	17	62.6	65	149.0	113	235.4	161	321.8	209	408.2
-30	-22.0	18	64.4	66	150.8	114	237.2	162	323.6	210	410.0
-29	-20.2	19	66.2	67	152.6	115	239.0	163	325.4	211	411.8
-28	-18.4	20	68.0	68	154.4	116	240.8	164	327.2	212	413.6
-27	-16.6	21	69.8	69	156.2	117	242.6	165	329.0	213	415.4
-26	-14.8	22	71.6	70	158.0	118	244.4	166	330.8	214	417.2
-25	-13.0	23	73.4	71	159.8	119	246.2	167	332.6	215	419.0
-24	-11.2	24	75.2	72	161.6	120	248.0	168	334.4	216	420.8
-23	- 9.4	25	77.0	73	163.4	121	249.8	169	336.2	217	422.6
-22	- 7.6	26	78.8	74	165.2	122	251.6	170	338.0	218	424.4
-21	- 5.8	27	80.6	75	167.0	123	253.4	171	339.8	219	426.2
-20	- 4.0	28	82.4	76	168.8	124	255.2	172	341.6	220	428.0
-19	- 2.2	29	84.2	77	170.6	125	257.0	173	343.4	221	429.8
-18	- 0.4	30	86.0	78	172.4	126	258.8	174	345.2	222	431.6
-17	+ 1.4	31	87.8	79	174.2	127	260.6	175	347.0	223	433.4
-16	3.2	32	89.6	80	176.0	128	262.4	176	348.8	224	435.2
-15	5.0	33	91.4	81	177.8	129	264.2	177	350.6	225	437.0
-14	6.8	34	93.2	82	179.6	130	266.0	178	352.4	226	438.8
-13	8.6	35	95.0	83	181.4	131	267.8	179	354.2	227	440.6
-12	10.4	36	96.8	84	183.2	132	269.6	180	356.0	228	442.4
-11	12.2	37	98.6	85	185.0	133	271.4	181	357.8	229	444.2
-10	14.0	38	100.4	86	186.8	134	273.2	182	359.6	230	446.0
- 9	15.8	39	102.2	87	188.6	135	275.0	183	361.4	231	447.8
- 8	17.6	40	104.0	88	190.4	136	276.8	184	363.2	232	449.6
- 7	19.4	41	105.8	89	192.2	137	278.6	185	365.0	233	451.4
- 6	21.2	42	107.6	90	194.0	138	280.4	186	366.8	234	453.2
- 5	23.0	43	109.4	91	195.8	139	282.2	187	368.6	235	455.0
- 4	24.8	44	111.2	92	197.6	140	284.0	188	370.4	236	456.8
- 3	26.6	45	113.0	93	199.4	141	285.8	189	372.2	237	458.6
- 2	28.4	46	114.8	94	201.2	142	287.6	190	374.0	238	460.4
- 1	30.2	47	116.6	95	203.0	143	289.4	191	375.8	239	462.2
0	32.0	48	118.4	96	204.8	144	291.2	192	377.6	240	464.0
+ 1	33.8	49	120.2	97	206.6	145	293.0	193	379.4	241	465.8
2	35.6	50	122.0	98	208.4	146	294.8	194	381.2	242	467.6
3	37.4	51	123.8	99	210.2	147	296.6	195	383.0	243	469.4
4	39.2	52	125.6	100	212.0	148	298.4	196	384.8	244	471.2
5	41.0	53	127.4	101	213.8	149	300.2	197	386.6	246	474.8
6	42.8	54	129.2	102	215.6	150	302.0	198	388.4	248	478.4
7	44.6	55	131.0	103	217.4	151	303.8	199	390.2	250	482.0

THERMOMETERS

Table for Conversion from Degrees Centigrade to Degrees Fahrenheit

Degrees Centigrade	0	10	20	30	40	50	60	70	80	90
					Degrees Fahrenheit					
−200	−328	−346	−364	−382	−400	−418	−436	−454	.....	.....
−100	−148	−166	−184	−202	−220	−238	−256	−274	−292	−310
−0	+32	+14	−4	−22	−40	−58	−76	−94	−112	−130
0	32	50	68	86	104	122	140	158	176	194
100	212	230	248	266	284	302	320	338	356	374
200	392	410	428	446	464	482	500	518	536	554
300	572	590	608	626	644	662	680	698	716	734
400	752	770	788	806	824	842	860	878	896	914
500	932	950	968	986	1004	1022	1040	1058	1076	1094
600	1112	1130	1148	1166	1184	1202	1220	1238	1256	1274
700	1292	1310	1328	1346	1364	1382	1400	1418	1436	1454
800	1472	1490	1508	1526	1544	1562	1580	1598	1616	1634
900	1652	1670	1688	1706	1724	1742	1760	1778	1796	1814
1000	1832	1850	1868	1886	1904	1922	1940	1958	1976	1994
1100	2012	2030	2048	2066	2084	2102	2120	2138	2156	2174
1200	2192	2210	2228	2246	2264	2282	2300	2318	2336	2354
1300	2372	2390	2408	2426	2444	2462	2480	2498	2516	2534
1400	2552	2570	2588	2606	2624	2642	2660	2678	2696	2714
1500	2732	2750	2768	2786	2804	2822	2840	2858	2876	2894
1600	2912	2930	2948	2966	2984	3002	3020	3038	3056	3074
1700	3092	3110	3128	3146	3164	3182	3200	3218	3236	3254
1800	3272	3290	3308	3326	3344	3362	3380	3398	3416	3434
1900	3452	3470	3488	3506	3524	3542	3560	3578	3596	3614
2000	3632	3650	3668	3686	3704	3722	3740	3758	3776	3794
2100	3812	3830	3848	3866	3884	3902	3920	3938	3956	3974
2200	3992	4010	4028	4046	4064	4082	4100	4118	4136	4154
2300	4172	4190	4208	4226	4244	4262	4280	4298	4316	4334
2400	4352	4370	4388	4406	4424	4442	4460	4478	4496	4514
2500	4532	4550	4568	4586	4604	4622	4640	4658	4676	4694
2600	4712	4730	4748	4766	4784	4802	4820	4838	4856	4874
2700	4892	4910	4928	4946	4964	4982	5000	5018	5036	5054
2800	5072	5090	5108	5126	5144	5162	5180	5198	5216	5234
2900	5252	5270	5288	5306	5324	5342	5360	5378	5396	5414
3000	5432	5450	5468	5486	5504	5522	5540	5558	5576	5594
3100	5612	5630	5648	5666	5684	5702	5720	5738	5756	5774
3200	5792	5810	5828	5846	5864	5882	5900	5918	5936	5954
3300	5972	5990	6008	6026	6044	6062	6080	6098	6116	6134
3400	6152	6170	6188	6206	6224	6242	6260	6278	6296	6314
3500	6332	6350	6368	6386	6404	6422	6440	6458	6476	6494
3600	6512	6530	6548	6566	6584	6602	6620	6638	6656	6674
3700	6692	6710	6728	6746	6764	6782	6800	6818	6836	6854
3800	6872	6890	6908	6926	6944	6962	6980	6998	7016	7034
3900	7052	7070	7088	7106	7124	7142	7160	7178	7196	7214
4000	7232	7250	7268	7286	7304	7322	7340	7358	7376	7394

Table for Converting Millimeters into Inches

Millimeters	Inches	Millimeters	Inches	Millimeters	Inches	Millimeters	Inches	Millimeters	Inches
1	0.0394	51	2.0079	101	3.9764	151	5.9450	201	7.9135
2	0.0787	52	2.0473	102	4.0158	152	5.9844	202	7.9529
3	0.1181	53	2.0867	103	4.0552	153	6.0237	203	7.9923
4	0.1575	54	2.1260	104	4.0946	154	6.0631	204	8.0316
5	0.1969	55	2.1654	105	4.1339	155	6.1025	205	8.0710
6	0.2362	56	2.2048	106	4.1733	156	6.1418	206	8.1104
7	0.2756	57	2.2441	107	4.2127	157	6.1812	207	8.1498
8	0.3150	58	2.2835	108	4.2520	158	6.2206	208	8.1891
9	0.3543	59	2.3229	109	4.2914	159	6.2600	209	8.2285
10	0.3937	60	2.3622	110	4.3308	160	6.2993	210	8.2679
11	0.4331	61	2.4016	111	4.3702	161	6.3387	211	8.3072
12	0.4724	62	2.4410	112	4.4095	162	6.3781	212	8.3466
13	0.5118	63	2.4804	113	4.4489	163	6.4174	213	8.3860
14	0.5512	64	2.5197	114	4.4883	164	6.4568	214	8.4253
15	0.5906	65	2.5591	115	4.5276	165	6.4962	215	8.4647
16	0.6299	66	2.5985	116	4.5670	166	6.5356	216	8.5041
17	0.6693	67	2.6378	117	4.6064	167	6.5749	217	8.5435
18	0.7087	68	2.6772	118	4.6458	168	6.6143	218	8.5828
19	0.7480	69	2.7166	119	4.6851	169	6.6537	219	8.6222
20	0.7874	70	2.7560	120	4.7245	170	6.6930	220	8.6616
21	0.8268	71	2.7953	121	4.7639	171	6.7324	221	8.7009
22	0.8662	72	2.8347	122	4.8032	172	6.7718	222	8.7403
23	0.9055	73	2.8741	123	4.8426	173	6.8111	223	8.7797
24	0.9449	74	2.9134	124	4.8820	174	6.8505	224	8.8191
25	0.9843	75	2.9528	125	4.9213	175	6.8899	225	8.8584
26	1.0236	76	2.9922	126	4.9607	176	6.9293	226	8.8978
27	1.0630	77	3.0316	127	5.0000	177	6.9686	227	8.9372
28	1.1024	78	3.0709	128	5.0394	178	7.0080	228	8.9765
29	1.1418	79	3.1103	129	5.0788	179	7.0474	229	9.0159
30	1.1811	80	3.1497	130	5.1182	180	7.0867	230	9.0553
31	1.2205	81	3.1890	131	5.1576	181	7.1261	231	9.0947
32	1.2599	82	3.2284	132	5.1969	182	7.1655	232	9.1340
33	1.2992	83	3.2678	133	5.2363	183	7.2049	233	9.1734
34	1.3386	84	3.3071	134	5.2757	184	7.2442	234	9.2128
35	1.3780	85	3.3465	135	5.3151	185	7.2836	235	9.2521
36	1.4173	86	3.3859	136	5.3544	186	7.3230	236	9.2915
37	1.4567	87	3.4253	137	5.3938	187	7.3623	237	9.3309
38	1.4961	88	3.4646	138	5.4332	188	7.4017	238	9.3702
39	1.5355	89	3.5040	139	5.4725	189	7.4411	239	9.4096
40	1.5748	90	3.5434	140	5.5119	190	7.4805	240	9.4490
41	1.6142	91	3.5827	141	5.5513	191	7.5198	241	9.4884
42	1.6536	92	3.6221	142	5.5907	192	7.5592	242	9.5277
43	1.6929	93	3.6615	143	5.6300	193	7.5986	243	9.5671
44	1.7323	94	3.7009	144	5.6694	194	7.6379	244	9.6065
45	1.7717	95	3.7402	145	5.7088	195	7.6773	245	9.6458
46	1.8111	96	3.7796	146	5.7481	196	7.7167	246	9.6852
47	1.8504	97	3.8190	147	5.7875	197	7.7560	247	9.7246
48	1.8898	98	3.8583	148	5.8269	198	7.7954	248	9.7640
49	1.9292	99	3.8977	149	5.8662	199	7.8348	249	9.8033
50	1.9685	100	3.9371	150	5.9056	200	7.8742	250	9.8427

INDEX

Become Younger

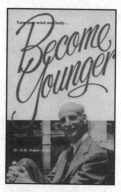

BECOME YOUNGER might be called the "cornerstone" of the famous Walker Program. What place has nutrition in the scheme of good health? How can the body and mind be so tuned that "old age" might be defeated? Dr. Walker suggests "When we embark on this program which may change our eating, drinking and living habits, we must have the courage of our convictions based on the knowledge which we can acquire through the principles involved in this program... To "become younger" means to have attained a state of sublime *self-reliance* and *self-sufficiency which no one can take away from us.*"

Colon Health

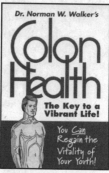

In COLON HEALTH Dr. Walker will take this forgotten part of your body and focus your full attention on it-and you'll never again take it for granted! This book shows how every organ, gland and cell in your body is affected by the condition of the large intestine-the colon. COLON HEALTH answers such questions as: Are cathartics and laxatives dangerous? - Can colon care prevent heart attack? - Is your eyesight affected by the condition of your colon? - What are the ghastly results of a colostomy?

Diet & Salad

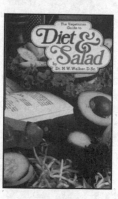

The pitfalls of overindulgence in certain food elements, especially oil and sugar, have been well documented. Dr. Walker offers in his book DIET & SALAD both a cookbook and a nutritional guide that belongs in every kitchen. In it he supports current medical research about the harmful effects of milk- "It is generally assumed that cow's milk is one of our most perfect foods...Milk is the most mucus forming food in the human diet, and it is the most insidious cause of colds, flu, bronchial troubles, asthma, hay fever, pneumonia, and sinus trouble...cow's milk was never intended for a human infant."

Fresh Vegetable and Fruit Juices

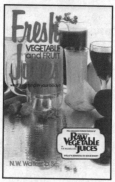

In FRESH VEGETABLE AND FRUIT JUICES, R. D. Pope, M.D., writes - "Dr. Walker has, for the first time in history, written a complete guide of the Therapeutic uses of our more common, everyday vegetables, when taken in the form of fresh, raw juices. It will be of considerable help to those who wish to derive the utmost benefit from the natural foods which God created for the nourishment of Man." Dr. Walker categorically lists vegetable juices, explains their elements, and in cooperation with Dr. Pope, provides suggestions for effective treatment of special ailments.

Vibrant Health

PROPER NUTRITION IS TANTAMOUNT TO GOOD HEALTH. One man today is walking proof of all this. Dr. NORMAN W. WALKER, a living example of VIBRANT HEALTH, has had the answer since 1910. His information is timeless. The originator of "juice therapy," he made this statement in the preface to one of his books: "The lack or deficiency of certain elements, such as vital organic minerals and salts, and consequently of vitamins, from our customary diet is the primary cause of nearly every sickness and disease." For three quarters of a century MEDICAL EVIDENCE HAS NOT REFUTED HIM.

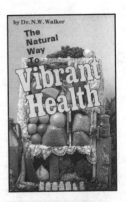

by Dr. N.W. Walker
The Natural Way To Vibrant Health

Water Can Undermine Your Health

Dr. Walker sees water pollution as a cause of arthritis, varicose veins, cancer, and even heart attacks- a major problem in virtually every community in the country. His treatment of water pollution is revealing, comprehensive, and scientific. His findings, and his recommendations for corrective action, offer new hope.

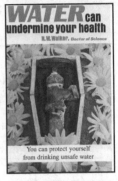

WATER can undermine your health
N.W. Walker, Doctor of Science

You can protect yourself from drinking unsafe water

Natural Weight Control

In NATURAL WEIGHT CONTROL, Dr. Walker offers "A Diet Like No Other"- based on the body's need for vital, life-giving enzymes found only in nature's pure foods. On enzymes he writes- "Enzymes are not things or substances! They are the life-principle in the atoms and molecules of every living cell. The enzymes in the cells of the human body are exactly like those in vegetation, and the atoms in the human body each have a corresponding affinity for like atoms in vegetation."

Easy Weight Control with NEW FOOD COMBINING PLAN

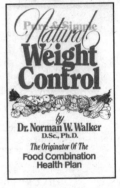

Pure & Simple Natural Weight Control
by Dr. Norman W. Walker D.Sc., Ph.D.
The Originator Of The Food Combination Health Plan

Educational Wall Charts

ENDOCRINE GLAND - See where they are located, their innumerable functions, what elements compose them, and what Juices nourish them.

COLON THERAPY- A most complete chart of the human Colon, indicating the relation of nerve endings from head to foot registered in the Colon, to alert you to your own condition.

FOOT RELAXATION - Shows Zones on the Soles of the Feet for use in relaxing tension in various parts of your body.

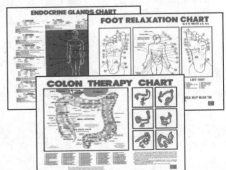

ENDOCRINE GLANDS CHART
FOOT RELAXATION CHART
COLON THERAPY CHART

NORWALK
PRESS

Year after year Modern Medical Science continues to prove Dr. Walker is right.

QTY.	TITLE	PRICE	TOTAL
	Diet and Salad	$9.95	
	Fresh Vegetables and Fruit Juices	$9.95	
	Vibrant Health	$9.95	
	Water Can Undermine Your Health	$9.95	
	Become Younger	$9.95	
	Colon Health	$9.95	
	Natural Weight Control	$9.95	
	Foot Relaxation Chart	$6.95	
	Colon Therapy Chart	$6.95	
	Endocrine Glands Chart	$6.95	
	Sub-Total		$
	___ items x $3.95 Each Item (S&H)		$
	TOTAL AMOUNT		$

NAME _____

STREET ADDRESS _____

CITY _____

STATE _____ ZIP _____

To order using this page please xerox the page, make your selection(s), and then calculate your total. Please send your xerox of this page and a check or money order to:

Mail Order Catalog • P.O. Box 180 • Summertown, TN 38483
1-800-695-2241

You may also purchase these health titles from your local bookstore or natural food store.

To find your favorite vegetarian and soyfood products online, visit: www.healthy-eating.com